Inside the Lion's Den

Inside the Lion's Den

Ken Shamrock
Richard Hanner

Principal photographer: Calixtro Romias

Charles E. Tuttle Co., Inc.
Boston • Rutland, Vermont • Tokyo

First published in 1998 by Tuttle Publishing, an imprint of Periplus Editions (HK) Ltd, with editorial offices at 153 Milk Street, Boston, Massachusetts 02109.

Library of Congress Cataloging-in-Publication Data

Shamrock 1964 –
    Inside the Lion's Den /Ken Shamrock, Richard Hanner: principle photographer, Clixtro Romias.
        p.   cm.
    ISBN 0-8048-3151-3 (pbk.)
    1. Shamrock, Ken, 1964 –. 2. Martial artists—United States—Biography. 3. Martial arts. I. Hanner, Richard. II. Romias, Calixtro. III. Title
GV1113.S53S53 1998
796.8' 092—dc21   97-45541
[B]   CIP

Distributed by

USA
Tuttle Publishing
Distribution Center
Airport Industrial Park
364 Innovation Drive
North Clarendon, VT 05759-9436
Tel: (802) 773-8930
Tel: (800) 526-2778

CANADA
Raincoast Books
8680 Cambie Street
Vancouver, British Columbia
V6P 6M9
Tel: (604) 323-7100
Fax: (604) 323-2600

JAPAN
Tuttle Shuppan
RK Building, 2nd Floor
2-13-10 Shimo-Meguro, Meguro-Ku
Tokyo 153 0064
Tel: (03) 5437-0171
Fax: (03) 5437-0755

SOUTHEAST ASIA
Berkeley Books Pte Ltd
5 Little Road #08-01
Singapore 536983
Tel: (65) 280-1330
Fax: (65) 280-6290

06 05 04 03 02 01 00   10 9 8 7 6 5 4 3

Printed in the United States

Dedication

To my father, who saved my life and allowed me to grow up and become the man I am today. To my beautiful wife, Tina, whose endless love and support have made my life special. And to our children, Ryan, Connor, Sean, and Fallon, who have made our lives complete.

—*K.S.*

For my wife, Judith Yukiko Hayashida, with love and gratitude.

—*R.H.*

Acknowledgments

My thanks to Kim Wood for inspiration in training. My Lion's Den fighters for believing. You are my second family. This includes Frank, Guy, Tra, Vernon, Jerry, and Pete. To Maurice Smith and Dan Freeman for helping us prepare for battle. To my good friend Richard Hanner, who knows more about me than anyone besides my family. Thanks for taking time from your family to help tell about Lion's Den. And to Calixtro Romias, for your artistry with a camera.

—*Ken Shamrock*

My sincere thanks to Ken Shamrock, who shared a remarkable life; to Bob Shamrock, for his friendship and encouragement in writing this book; to Tina Shamrock, for her help and insight; to the Lion's Den fighters, who spent hours patiently telling me about their teacher, themselves, and submissions fighting (with special thanks to Frank Shamrock, Jerry Bohlander, Vernon White, and Pete Williams); to Calixtro Romias for his artistic vision; and to Curtis Glenn for creative counsel. I am indebted to Mark V. Wiley for both his nimble editing and great patience. I am also grateful to Robert Meyrowitz and his associates at Semaphore Entertainment Group, and Art Davie, commissioner of the International Fighting Council, who helped me understand the evolution of the Ultimate Fighting Championship.

—*Richard Hanner*

Table of Contents

PART TWO: INSIDE THE LION'S DEN

Foreword

In the autumn of 1993, it was announced that a local man, Ken Shamrock, was competing in a televised no-holds-barred fighting event. According to a press release, Shamrock was a submission fighter with a background in street brawling. I was assigned to do a feature story on Shamrock, a story I thought would be a routine piece, a profile of a dull brute of a man who had signed up for something called the Ultimate Fighting Championship. The story turned out to be no routine assignment.

I found myself intrigued by Shamrock's explanation of submission fighting and by his martial arts exploits in Japan. Even more, I was fascinated by his background, by his triumph over personal demons that might have destroyed him but did not.

After that interview, Shamrock quickly emerged as one of the most feared and respected martial artists of his generation. And as practiced by Shamrock at his Lion's Den dojo, submission fighting gained recognition as among the most formidable martial systems ever devised.

This book would be incomplete as mere biography; likewise, it would be lacking as simply an instructional manual.

So it is both.

Part One, Enter the Lion, explores Shamrock, a fighter, a son, a husband, a father. Part Two, Inside the Lion's Den, discusses submission fighting, the martial art Ken popularized and used to dominate no-holds-barred competition circuit.

I hope the following pages portray the warrior as fully and vividly as his style of hand-to-hand combat.

—*Richard Hanner*
Woodbridge, California

Enter the Lion

The Story of a Modern Gladiator

by Richard Hanner

Chapter 1

Lord of the Octagon

Detroit
Cobo Arena
May 17, 1996

K en Shamrock, the first King of Pancrase, three-time Ultimate Fighting Superfight Champion, winner of numerous bar brawls and Toughman wars, widely regarded as the finest no-holds-barred fighter in the world, is being booed.

Shamrock struts through an artificial mist into Cobo Arena, surrounded by his entourage of young gladiators. Above the procession waves the crimson flag of Lion's Den, the elite dojo where Shamrock trains the fiercest hand-to-hand fighters in the world. Shamrock's father, Bob Shamrock, hefts the Superfight champion's belt, a leather-and-brass trophy carrying the image of a man with a shaved head and massive, menacing fists.

Shamrock moves deeper into Cobo. And the malice of 12,000 Michiganders, many with guts bloated with beer, showers upon him. A paper tray of nachos explodes at the feet of the reigning king of the UFC as he approaches the octagon, the eight-sided fighting pit. "Chump!," screams the beer-lit man who tossed the cheesy bomb. "You're nothing but a big chump!"

Shamrock does not blink. He strides past the garbage, through the catcalls and howls rising from the throats of the rabid thousands, the legion who crave his blood tonight. Spotlights swirl around Shamrock like huge, incessant fireflies. Shamrock steps gracefully into the black-trimmed combat zone and sheds his satin yellow robe emblazoned with the name "Lion's Den." As the robe is pulled away, Shamrock's bronzed shoulders and arms and chest are revealed. His is the smoothly muscled torso of a Greek god.

Kenneth Wayne Shamrock is not a man easily shaken. He has fought many times in bars and alleys. He has hurt men too drunk or stupid to realize his powers. He has fought in Toughman contests staged in rodeo arenas and knocked men cold with a single lightning strike to the jaw. He has fought in the glittering Budokan martial arts

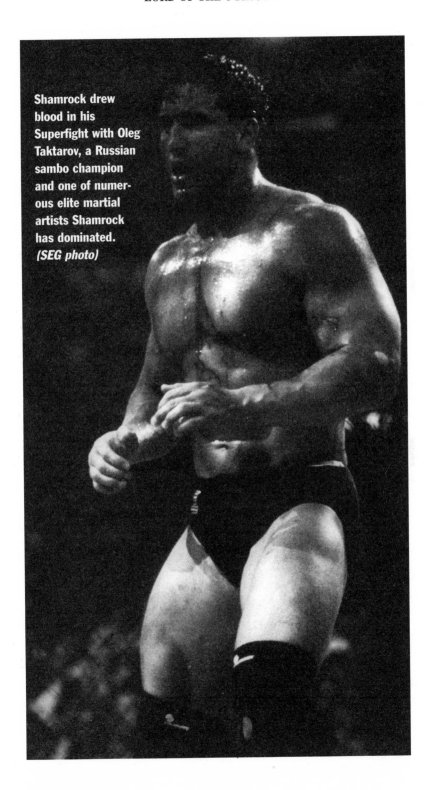

Shamrock drew blood in his Superfight with Oleg Taktarov, a Russian sambo champion and one of numerous elite martial artists Shamrock has dominated. *(SEG photo)*

dome in Tokyo, earning the first Pancrase belt. And he has fought in this octagon, in Denver and Charlotte and Buffalo and Casper and Puerto Rico, before millions of fans who pay $20 per TV set to see the raw blend of courage and carnage that is the Ultimate Fighting Championship (UFC).

Tonight, though, it will be different for the most dangerous man on the planet. Tonight, there is more, much more, on the line. There is a substantial purse, reportedly into six figures, that will do much to help secure his family's future. Shamrock has three young children. His wife, Tina, sitting only a few feet from the rust-spattered octagon, carries their unborn daughter inside her. Also ringside are the Hollywood people, the people who flew into Detroit this afternoon and know a victory tonight will help sell movie tickets in the months and years to come.

But there is, above all, the belt with the brass shield. The belt he has bled and bloodied for, the belt he must, if he wishes to cement his legend, retain here tonight.

Now bouncing gently, rhythmically, inside the fighting cage, Shamrock is an aging warrior. At 32, Shamrock's body is still sculpted

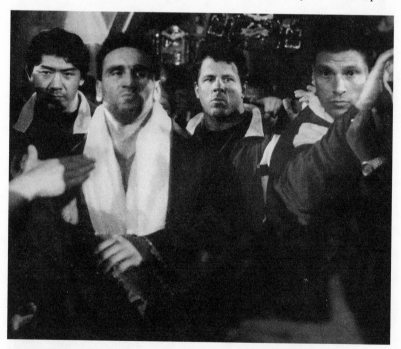

As Ken Shamrock entered Cobo Arena for his Superfight with Dan Severn, few in the audience realized the pressure he was under. (Calixtro Romias photo)

and powerful, but the infrastructure has suffered mightily from a lifetime of physical combat. Nose, jaw, neck, ribs, sternum—all have been broken. The hand has been fractured, the knee shattered. Shamrock does not know, cannot know, which battle will be his last.

Now Shamrock aims his hazel eyes across the octagon, directly into the eyes of Dan Severn, a mustachioed 270-pound wrestler. The two have fought before, in UFC XI in Wyoming. Shamrock, showing the submission technique he learned in Japan, quickly choked and toppled the giant. But Severn is a cunning and veteran warrior. He has studied Shamrock since the defeat, carefully analyzing his craft and art. After he lost to Shamrock, Severn fought in an event called the "Ultimate Ultimate," a tournament of martial arts champions from all over the globe. Showing bearish strength and ferocity, Severn prevailed as the tournament champion. Now, he is pumped, confident, thirsting for revenge. And Dan "The Beast" Severn, who lives in Coldwater, Michigan, is the hometown boy igniting Cobo tonight. He turns to the crowd, the largest live gate in the history of the UFC, and raises his massive arms toward the rafters. The crowd begins a deafening chant: "BEAST! BEAST! BEAST!"

A sheen of sweat rises from Shamrock's chest as John McCarthy, the Los Angeles cop and no-nonsense referee, steps to the center of the octagon. McCarthy is a big man dressed all in black, with writing on the back of his smock: "Who Is The World's Greatest Fighter?"

McCarthy looks at Severn. "Are you ready?," he asks. Severn nods. McCarthy wheels to Shamrock. "Are you ready?," he again asks. Shamrock tilts his jaw. "Okay," McCarthy yells, then slaps his fists together. "Let's get it on!"

As the combatants circle one another, the Detroit partisans stand, stomp their feet, and bellow like a frenzied herd: "BEAST! BEAST! BEAST!" And Cobo Arena quakes with a deafening, primordial pulse, the thunder of a crowd primed and ready for gladiatorial combat.

For the most dangerous fighter on the planet, things will be different tonight. There is something happening in Cobo tonight that no one expected.

Especially Ken Shamrock.

• • •

As the millennium ends, a new sport is being born. It is a sport with an ancient lineage, a lineage traced to the Greeks who faced each other in hand-to-hand combat called pankration. This contemporary sport has risen simultaneously in various corners of the earth: in Japan, in Brazil, in Russia, in the United States. The sport carries different names. Some, in deference to the Greeks, call it pankration. In Brazil, it is called vale tudo, for "anything goes." In the United States, it is called reality combat or no-holds-barred fighting.

Its critics simply call it barbaric.

These critics have tried to ban the newborn athletic event, ignoring the talent and skill and heart of those who compete in it, ignoring the fact that it descends from the Greeks, the people who best personify Western civilization. And despite efforts to ban reality fighting as being unworthy of a civilized society, it flourishes. Some maintain it is the essence of the martial arts, which they believe have grown too slick, too commercial. Others believe it is the essence of professional sports, of skilled men battling not only for money, but for honor.

Those who view the best examples of this new sport see splendid athletes, some of whom have studied their art longer than the most popular professional football or basketball players. They see these athletes compete in raw and ferocious contests that are nonetheless marvels of strategy and technique. The fights are mixtures of karate, judo, ju-jitsu, kickboxing, wrestling. Perhaps most prominently, they feature a martial system known as submission fighting, a well-rounded system that emphasizes the chokes and joint locks that defined pankration in the days of the Greeks.

And at the end of the millennium, a single man has risen to dominate this sport, this grueling test of muscle and mind and spirit.

His name is Kenneth Wayne Shamrock.

Shamrock has a history as a brawler and street fighter. But he tempered his fighting style in the dojos and fighting arenas of Japan, where he adopted and refined submission techniques. Competing in the Pancrase Hybrid Wrestling circuit, he quickly became one of the first *gaijin*, or foreigners, to win a Japanese fighting crown. Later, he won glory as the first Superfight champion of the Ultimate Fighting Championship, the most popular reality fighting contest in the United States.

As he ascended to the pinnacle of the sport, he faced the best of the competition and prevailed.

He choked out the Pancrase founder and Japanese fighting hero Masami Funaki.

He used a submission hold to defeat Bas Rutten, the Dutch fighting champion.

He dominated Royce Gracie, the pride of the Gracies of Brazil, a highly respected family of fighters which has developed its own formidable style of ju-jitsu.

He bloodied and bruised Oleg Taktarov, a national Russian sambo champion.

In his first fight with Severn, he choked and silenced him in less than three minutes.

And he wrenched the leg of the powerful fighter Kimo Leopoldo, forcing him to slam the canvas and proclaim his defeat.

Shamrock is the epitome of the modern gladiator. He is a singular fusion of agility and power and athletic grace. Lying on his back, Shamrock can hoist 600 pounds of iron over his chest. He can slam-dunk a basketball. He can drive a golf ball 350 yards. He can spar fiercely and without pause for an hour without getting winded. At six feet tall and 215 pounds, his body is hard and tight, like that of a giant cat. Shamrock is a sleek predator.

Beyond his physical talents are the gifts of the mind. Shamrock seems to sense movement before it happens. As a college linebacker, he penetrated so swiftly, so decisively, other teams thought he was eavesdropping on their play calls. As a no-holds-barred warrior, he has an unfailing sense of balance, of distance, of rhythm. Innately, Shamrock knows just how far to strike in order to rock the jaw of an opponent. He knows how high and fast to revolve behind an adversary to "sink in" a choke. How to deftly capture a leg rocketing at his ribs, seize it, and crank it until it threatens to be twisted off its owner, like a drumstick wrested from a chicken. Researchers call what Shamrock possesses kinesthetic intelligence.

Ken Shamrock is not a college graduate, but he is a genius of forceful movement.

He also has an uncanny ability to concentrate, to focus, to summon all of his formidable energies and reduce them to a single purpose, like a drill bit gnawing into lumber.

And he possesses something else, though it is not properly described as a gift. Shamrock has a blinding, burning rage. As much as athletic talent, as much as balletic technique, it is rage that has that has driven Shamrock. And it is rage that has nearly destroyed him.

Chapter 2

The Lion's Den

Lodi, California
March 10, 1996

The sinewy left arm of Ken Shamrock is slithering its way dangerously close to the neck of Vernon White. White tries valiantly to shove the powerful limb away. Yet it continues slipping, like some relentless viper, across the sternum, closer, closer to the vital pipeline that carries blood and oxygen to the brain of Vernon White. "Errrggg," White gurgles. He tears harder at Shamrock's arm, but it is now attacking just below White's Adam's apple, tightening like a rope, steady and sure and taut.

This is part of the day's work at the Lion's Den, the most successful and demanding gladiatorial dojo in America. Though the public is invited to take self-defense classes at the Lion's Den in the evening, these afternoon sessions are not open to the public. Shamrock closed the work-outs after some who viewed them grew revolted and accused Shamrock of brutality. Shamrock sees it much differently. He wants his fighters to be prepared. He wants his fighters to be victorious. "Marine boot camp is not fun. It is not pretty," says Shamrock, who has been there. "That's because they are preparing you for war. I am preparing my fighters for war."

Shamrock is lodged firmly behind White. A favorable place for Shamrock, a position of crisis for White. White is unfortunate in this respect as well: his tutor is training for what may be the toughest fight of his life, a rematch against Dan "The Beast" Severn. It is likely to be a grueling and nasty fight. Shamrock is not in a generous mood this afternoon.

Shamrock, in effect, is presenting another seminar for his warriors-in-training: advanced rear choke. White, though learning a painful lesson, is learning nonetheless. And the other fighters arrayed around the ring are learning as well. Shamrock has hand-picked each one of them, chosen them to be his elite, his fighting family. Lion's Den fighters have dominated reality competition all over the world. They have claimed victory in the UFC, in Pancrase, in the Superbrawl

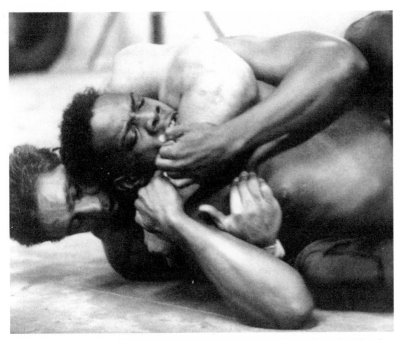

Shamrock is a demanding coach and mentor. Here he works relentlessly for a rear choke during training with Lion's Den fighter Vernon White. (Calixtro Romias photo)

in Hawaii, and the Vale Tudo Open in Brazil. The young fighters do not learn their craft from textbooks. They do not learn it doing kata, or the repetitive movements that help define some martial arts schools. They learn it by fighting, fighting with heart and soul and tenacity, in this space.

Some of the finest, most successful fighters in the world have trained here: Shamrock's brother, Frank Shamrock, who won a share of the Pancrase crown after training a little more than a year; Oleg Taktarov, "The Russian Bear," a sambo specialist and UFC veteran, a gutsy man who seems oblivious to pain; Jerry Bohlander, a UFC lightweight champion and Superbrawl champion; Maurice Smith, world heavyweight kickboxing, UFC and Extreme Fighting champion; Guy Mezger, a UFC and kickboxing champion; Tra Telligman, a super heavyweight champion in Hawaii and Russia, and Vernon White, a young Pancrase fighter and former karate practitioner.

Combined, Lion's Den fighters have won more no-holds-barred professional contests than fighters from any other dojo in the world.

Shamrock started the Lion's Den nearly a decade ago. The name,

Shamrock said, reflects the lion's ferocity and predatory skill. It also reflects the lion's instinct to hunt and survive as a pride, as a family.

There is no sign outside the Lion's Den. It is a clean and spartan place in an industrial area of Lodi, a city of 55,000 located in the great, fertile Central Valley of California. Shamrock has been asked to relocate to Southern California or New York, to be closer to the media, closer to the population masses that might turn his dojo into a golden sweatshop. He has refused. Lodi, a tidy town founded by German farmers and merchants, is free of distractions, free of glitz, a good place to raise a family. A good place too, to raise a family of earnest hand-to-hand warriors.

Inside the Lion's Den, there are high ceilings and wrestling mats neatly arranged on the floor. A rat's nest of jump ropes hangs from one wall, along with UFC promotional posters of Shamrock, glaring at opponents Gracie and Severn. There is a small refrigerator holding bottled water. Some of the fighters stow their protein drinks here as well. There is no water fountain here, and there are no showers. The refrigerator sits on a table holding copies of *Black Belt* magazines,

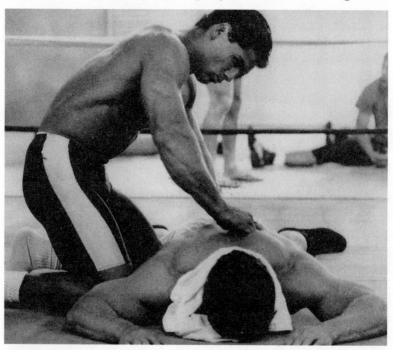

Frank Shamrock, who claimed a share of the Pancrase crown after just six months training at the Lion's Den, gives a rubdown to Ken Shamrock. (Calixtro Romias photo)

most of them a year or two old.

At the center of this place is an expanse of blue canvas over particle board, framed by corduroy-sleeved ropes. The canvas is scuffed and frayed. Close inspection reveals little puddles of rust, the dried remnants of combat. This ring is Shamrock's laboratory, his classroom. It is here that he reveals the secrets of his fighting system, submissions, to his acolytes.

The arm is twined securely around White's neck now. Shamrock is steadily tightening the hold, a steely vise around human flesh. The flow of air to White's brain is slowing, slowing. With a last furious spasm, White tries to tap out, slapping his hand against the mat. He even manages a whisper: "taaaap, tap - tap out!" He is a man at sea, sinking to the depths. But the tutor will not abandon today's lesson until it is completed. "No," Shamrock says. "No tap out." White's eyelashes flutter softly. Then his eyes are closed. The choke, in the parlance of the ring, is sunk in. Vernon White is unconscious.

Rear chokes, guillotine chokes, leg chokes, knee bars, and Achilles locks. Such is the curricula of submission warfare that is taught and mastered in the Lion's Den. Submission fighting has its roots in antiquity and Shamrock readily admits that he didn't invent the system; he only refined it, tempered it in various battles, pushed it to a higher level. Submission fighting was actually invented by the Greeks, who used it in their pancration event, a blend of striking and grappling. Pancration had no time limit; the struggle lasted until one of the combatants gave up. The only prohibitions were eye gouging and biting. These minimal rules were strictly enforced by a referee who used a stick to flog violators until they complied. With its blend of strikes, kicks, and technically demanding holds, the pankration drew the toughest, most skilled fighters to the ancient Olympics, along with the largest, most vociferous crowds. Pancration fighters, able to fight on their feet as well as the ground, were revered above all other martial combatants.

Shamrock's submissions system does not stress the spiritual element that defines some Eastern martial arts. It is purely a fighting art, aggressive and pragmatic, and its adherents do not meditate or burn incense. Submissions, stark and technical, is not the stuff of which a fanciful television series would be made. And while Shamrock studies and fights regularly in Japan, and has for six years, he does not attempt to transfer Asian cultural or spiritual traditions to his dojo. "This is not Japan," he sometimes tells his fighters. "And we are not Japanese."

In his dojo, Shamrock does not encourage his students to call him *sensei*, for master, though some refer to him simply as "king," a reference to the King of Pancrase title Shamrock won in 1995. The business of the Lion's Den is submission fighting, and it is carried out with all the frill and pomp one might find in a high school metal shop.

It is Shamrock, more than any contemporary martial artist, who has shown the grace and efficiency of submission fighting. He has shown, too, the need to fuse both striking and grappling skills, to continually revise and refine one's art. His main proving ground has been the UFC, the breakthrough mixed-martial arts event first staged in 1993. Before national television audiences, Shamrock has faced and beaten judo, karate, taekwondo, and kickboxing champions. Shamrock has moved beyond punches, chops, and reverse kicks. He has improved and developed the groundwork, subtle and demanding, that usually decides a no-holds-barred rumble. "By showing the importance of grappling, Ken has helped revolutionize the martial arts," says Art Davie, Ultimate Fighting Championship commissioner. Davie, a former U.S. Marine and amateur boxer, rates Shamrock with Royce Gracie and Bruce Lee as the most influential martial artists in the last twenty years. "Ken has evolved better than anyone else who has fought in the UFC."

White's descent is neither an isolated nor unexpected occurrence in the Lion's Den. Each fighter has drawn blood, been bloodied, choked and been choked out. "Vernon go night-night," observes Bohlander, sitting just a few feet away, as White slips under. Shamrock withdraws his arm, but stays close to White, leaning over him. With Shamrock's chokehold released, White's lungs pump a surge of oxygen to his brain, and slowly, his body reawakens. "Wha, wha, where am I?," he asks. "Hey Vernon, you've been sleeping on the job," offers Bohlander.

"Keep fighting," Shamrock demands. White's eyes reopen. He is still groggy, but Shamrock moves above him, grinding his weight into White's chest. "We're not done yet," Shamrock says. White rolls his hips and tries to flip his mentor away. He fails. For another minute, Shamrock rocks his weight on White, and White tries futilely to resist. Then, satisfied his lesson has been absorbed, Shamrock pushes away from White and rises.

When the modern Olympics began in 1906, boxing and wrestling were revived but pankration was not. It is possible that tales of the pankration's brutality prevented its resurrection. Olympic historians, for instance, say that one pancration champion was strangled in 564

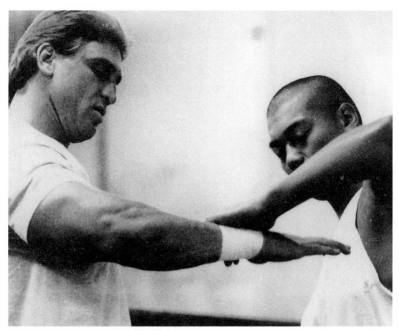

At the Lion's Den, the rookies, known as young boys, serve the established fighters. Here Haygar Chin wraps the wrist of Ken Shamrock.
Calixtro Romias photo

as he won the event for the third time. Before he died, the fighter managed to break the toes of his rival and forced him to tap out. So the man, even in death, was hailed as a hero.

When the Romans adopted pankration, they added bladed gloves. Competitors slashed and mutilated one another. Pankration, begun as the essence of athleticism, devolved into pure bloodsport. It is the art of submission fighting created by the Greeks that Shamrock has used so convincingly in the Ultimate Fighting Championship. It is the art now practiced each day in a simple, unmarked space in Lodi, California. Practiced, and also revised. A new angle for a choke, a slightly different grip for an kneebar, can always be found. Submission fighting, Lion's Den style, is as old as the ancient Greeks but as new as the last work-out.

As he towels off, Shamrock underlines his teaching approach. "My fighters face a lot more here than they do in the octagon or anywhere else," he says. "We push to the limit. And then we push some more."

In the long term, Shamrock maintains, the beatings and breakdowns endured in this gray-walled chamber eventually lead to mental and physical toughening. The toughening leads to confidence. And the confidence leads to success. "I don't want my fighters losing. And I don't want them getting injured. I want them to go into a fight ready for anything. People don't see that. They just don't understand."

It is best, Shamrock knows, to go after his fighters hard and rough, with no holds barred, no quarter given. It is the same way, he knows, that Dan "The Beast" Severn will come after him.

Shamrock, when he fights at Cobo Arena in less than ninety days, must be ready for war.

Chapter 3

Roots of Rage

Savannah, Georgia
1969

T
he brothers were under attack. Pelted, chased, shoved to the ground. Even their home was no refuge. The others simply stormed in through the windows, continued the assault, stole what they wanted.

Early childhood is the time, say researchers, when personality, outlook, and attitude are shaped. Early childhood was the time when Ken Shamrock learned to fight. It is also the period when the rage

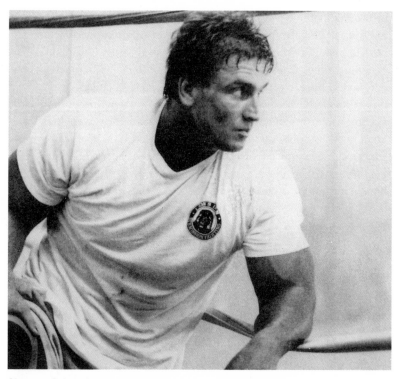

Shamrock has learned to subdue the rage that nearly consumed him as a youth. *(Calixtro Romias photo)*

grew inside of him, the rage that would both drive him—and threaten to devour him.

The roots of this rage lie in the red clay of Georgia, where Shamrock was born and lived for the first four years of his life. Shamrock was born Kenneth Wayne Kilpatrick in the hospital at the Warner Robins Air Force Base. His father was Richard Kilpatrick, a fast-talking former Air Force enlistee who left the military to use his gift of gab peddling shoes. Kilpatrick was a ne'er-do-well and a lady's man. Shamrock's mother was Diane Kilpatrick, an attractive but compliant woman who loved her children but had no a clue how to discipline them. Shamrock had two older brothers, Richie and Robbie. Soon after Shamrock was born, the family moved from Warner-Robbins to Savannah, where his father drifted further and further from the family. Finally, Richard Kilpatrick wasn't even living in the same house, though he would sometimes stop by, according to relatives, and pilfer checks from his estranged wife.

Diane, who had her first son at age fifteen, was left to provide for her three boys by herself. It was a challenge that nearly overwhelmed the young mother. She took jobs as a waitress and dancer at a club in Savannah.The babysitters she hired were less than diligent, leaving the boys to look after themselves, to run wild in the streets of a subsidized housing project. Each of the boys remember the neighborhood as being dominated by African-Americans. And each remembers being regularly attacked by other youngsters, most of them bigger and older. Richie Kilpatrick recalls hurling a brick at a boy who had tossed Shamrock to the ground and was pounding on him. The brick drew a gusher of blood and a series of reprisal ambushes. "We had kids climbing through the windows to get at us," Richie Kilpatrick recalls. "It was like being under attack. We had to close the windows and lock the doors." (Though Shamrock recalls feeling isolated as a youngster because of his race, he has grown into a man who embraces all races and cultures. The Lion's Den has featured fighters of African-American, Hispanic and Asian backgrounds; all are welcome.)

One of Shamrock's earliest memories is of his kindergarten teacher grabbing him and pulling him toward the principal's office by his earlobe. Shamrock slugged the woman in the stomach, then sprinted to the classroom and locked the door, alone and seething. He was eventually extracted from his refuge, yelping and thrashing, and taken home.

When the Kilpatrick boys weren't skirmishing with other children, they wandered, going through dumpsters, exploring back alleys and vacant lots. "We'd look for food, look for toys. Whatever we could find," Richie Kilpatrick recalled. "We learned to fend for ourselves. Survival was in our blood at any early age."

Beyond the time he slugged the teacher, Shamrock remembers little of these formative years. The memories are of the constant fighting, the bruising ambushes and harassment by other youngsters. If in the early years of Shamrock's youth there were Christmas mornings with ornaments and gifts, if there were birthday cakes and candles, those images have faded. What remains are the vivid scenes of conflict. Of fighting to survive. "About all I had was my pride. And it seemed the other kids were trying to grab that away from me. So I fought," Shamrock said. "We all fought."

When Shamrock was five, Diane Kilpatrick, divorced from Richard Kilpatrick, married an Army aviator named Bob Nance. The hastily constructed family moved to Napa, California, Nance's hometown. Napa is a comfortable community tucked in the scenic and prosperous California wine country. But here, too, the boys felt like outsiders. They were from a poor background, they spoke in a Georgia drawl and they had the hardened attitude of alley cats. The fighting continued, but the boys also started stealing and experimenting with drugs.

Nance, a driven and determined man, left the Army and joined the Napa fire department. He also worked as a roofer and upholsterer. Nance knew nothing about raising kids and little about reaching out to young people. He'd seen good friends wounded and killed in Vietnam. He dealt with suffering and death frequently as a firefighter. Though he cared for the three young hooligans who were now his stepsons, he was not emotionally equipped to nurture or direct them. "I could never be a counselor or a psychotherapist. I just don't have the patience for that," he said. Nance tried to steer his young charges toward sports, hoping the structure of Little League and Pop Warner football might help tame them. Shamrock, in fact, became a star in the Napa Pop Warner league. "I had one veteran coach come up to me at the awards banquet and say he'd never seen a football player with as much heart and tenacity as Kenny," Nance said. "Even then, Kenny was a remarkable athlete." Shamrock avoided drugs, but his brother Robbie remembers enjoying both marijuana and football. "I was a stoner jock," he said.

Despite the constructive exposure to sports, the boys continued to resist and rebel. They'd brawl at school, steal Twinkies from the corner market, hustle younger kids for lunch money. Nance dealt with it the only way he knew how: with steely militaristic discipline. "If one of us stole something, Bob would march us inside. He'd line us up and make us drop our pants. Then he'd whip our butts with the belt until one of us confessed," Richie Kilpatrick said. "Bob tried with us, he really did. He just didn't know how to be a loving dad." As adults, all three boys now say they respect Nance and appreciate what he was up against. "I don't think Bob Nance knew what he was getting into when he married our mom," Robbie Kilpatrick said. "He tried to be our father, but I looked at him and thought 'he's not our father, why does he think he can boss us around?' There was a time I hated Bob Nance. I think I ran away from home just to get away from him."

Shamrock remembers the household as being emotionally charged, pressurized, volcanic. "There was a lot of yelling and whipping. Bob had a military background. He wanted to control us, but we loved our freedom. We didn't want to be controlled." The boys resented Nance, this seemingly cold man so quick to unfurl his belt. They started running away from home, living with friends in abandoned cars or shacks. Shamrock remembers leaving home for the first time at age ten. He lived in an abandoned car with some other kids for a few days, subsisting on munchies he shoplifted from a local convenience store. After being stabbed by an older kid, Shamrock wound up in the hospital. Doctors contacted youth justice officials and Shamrock found himself in juvenile hall for the first time. He remembers the lock-up as oddly relaxing. "I didn't mind it. Compared to home, it was quiet and rather peaceful," Shamrock said.

Bob Nance's return to Napa marked the beginning of some of the most trying and turbulent years of his life. His new stepsons, rapidly approaching adolescence, were defiant young hellions. There were numerous late-night trips to the police station and hospital to pick up one or more of the boys. His lashings with both tongue and belt had an immediate but short-lived impact. "As soon as I'd leave, they'd go back to raising hell," he said. "So I'd come home and beat the crap out of them again." Diane Kilpatrick, who passed away in 1995, was little help. She was nearly phobic about confrontation. "There'd be a knockdown, drag-out fight going on in the house, and my mom would be sitting in a chair, reading a book," Shamrock recalled.

Finally, Nance's patience was spent. He'd signed the boys up for sports, watched as many of the games as his relentless schedule permitted. He'd made a point to take the boys camping and to bring them to firemen's musters, where firefighters compete in events such as racing or climbing with heavy hoses. He'd worked three jobs to provide for his family. All, it seemed, to no avail.

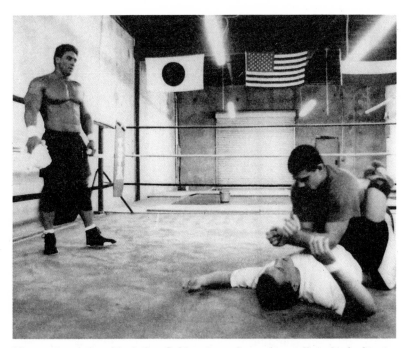

Shamrock requires Lion's Den fighters to undergo demanding physical tests before they can enter his dojo. Two aspirants who made the grade are Pete Williams and Jerry Bohlander (on his back). *(Calixtro Romias photo)*

So in 1977, the young stepfather took a drastic step. "I just told them 'you don't live here anymore.' I notified the police and juvenile authorities that the boys were on the street. I just wasn't going to take it anymore."

Ken Shamrock was thirteen years old at the time.

The three brothers went their separate ways. Each would be scarred by these early years of chaos and conflict. Each would have their brushes with the law. Each would do time in juvenile lock-ups and one would do time in the state penitentiary.

But one would later take the name Shamrock. And become a husband, a father, and one of the most celebrated hand-to-hand warriors of his generation.

Chapter 4

The Test

Lodi
May 24, 1996

F irst, you have to pass the test, even then, I can only take one, maybe two."

Shamrock stands before the tense young men, the young hopefuls, assembled inside Lion's Den. They have come from all over the United States and Canada. The age range is nineteen to twenty-six.

Some, like Craig, who rode a Greyhound bus for three days from a village in Canada, are tall and lean. A few, like Ron, from a city just to the south of Lodi, are solid and layered with muscle. All have wrestling, martial arts, or heavy street fighting experience. There are six of them standing before Shamrock this afternoon, six stalwarts trying out for the most exclusive fighting dojo in the country. They believe they are prepared for this test. But they have no idea. The next two hours will be among the most hellish in their lives.

Shamrock steps in front of them. "Most of you will give up," he announces. "That doesn't mean you are less of a man. And it doesn't mean you can't try again. Not many guys are good enough or tough enough to even attempt this. Good luck to all of you."

The heat is building in the Lion's Den on this spring afternoon. There is no air conditioning. The big steel roll-up door has been opened in hopes a cooling breeze might rise from the nearby Delta, but the air remains warm and still.

Those chosen today, those who survive, will toil and suffer in this place. Bleed into the blue canvas of the ring. Maybe weep into it as well. When they have completed their course, which will take six months or longer, they will be among the toughest, best-rounded fighters in the world. They will be capable of pumping hundreds of squats and push-ups in secession, sparring for an hour without stopping, and choking out their prey with the efficiency of a boa constrictor crushing a rat.

While in training, the fighters live in a rural home owned by Shamrock. They eat chicken breasts and rice bought with

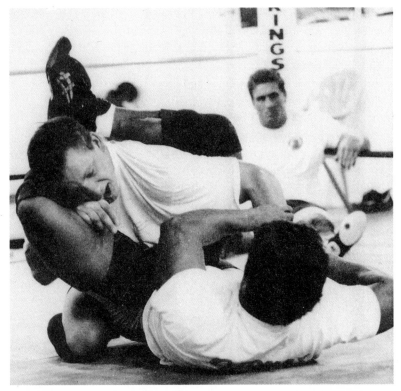

Those who become Lion's Den fighters receive personal coaching from Shamrock, here watching Jerry Bohlander working in the guard of Frank Shamrock. *(Calixtro Romias photo)*

Shamrock's money. They train when Shamrock tells them to train, fight when he tells them to fight. They will do the scut work in the fighter's home, broiling chicken breasts for the veterans, cleaning the toilets, vacuuming the rugs. It is like Marine boot camp, a process of breaking down to build up. "When I joined the dojo, the first thing Ken did was beat me up," recalls Frank. "He just beat the living crap out of me. He beats you down and shows you that you aren't as bad and as tough as you think you are. He takes all that selfish ego away. And then he starts giving you something back. He tells you that you will be a fighter. And he shows you how. If you stick with it, you become a fighter, maybe a great one." After just a year of training with Lion's Den, Frank Shamrock became one of the top fighters with the Pancrase Hybrid Wrestling association in Japan.

For the fighters, the blandishments are varied. First is money: the young men may earn $60,000 or $80,000 or more per year on a fighting circuit. With a few victories, they will be treated with the same respect as any professional athlete. They will be asked to pose for photos with the arms of perfect strangers draped over their shoulders. They will be asked to write their names on pieces of papers and T-shirts and brochures and photos and these inky scribbles will be treasured by their owners.

After a fighter has transcended the status of the young boy, there remain the expectations of training and fighting with a gladiator's heart. Otherwise, there are few pressures. The fighters often lounge or swim or play volleyball during their off-hours. They stay up late at night, often until 1 AM, watching films of no-holds combat or noisily battling one another in video games. "We suffer from an acute lack of responsibility," said veteran fighter Jerry Bohlander, only half-jokingly.

In exchange for this lifestyle, and for the chicken breasts and rice and the fighting secrets he provides, Shamrock gets ten percent of the fighters' winnings for five years. There are plans to start Lion's Den training and fighting centers in other cities. Some of the fighters will be asked to supervise them.

There are no advertisements for the try-out today. It is by invitation only. If Shamrock has seen videotape of you and you looked good and tough enough, you might get a shot. If you've worked out at the self-defense classes Shamrock offers at the Lion's Den twice a week, and you've shown some muscle and heart, you might be asked to participate.

For the first stage of the test, the fighters must leave the dojo. A caravan of vehicles rumbles from Lion's Den to a Lodi-area high school. The high school's football stadium is the first testing ground. The proctors for this examination are Shamrock's resident fighters, including Frank Shamrock, Vernon White, Jerry Bohlander, and Haygar Chin. The afternoon sun is growing intense now, and each of the well-muscled fighters has stripped to his shorts. Shamrock calls his assistants into a huddle, away from the aspirants. "I don't want any profanity. No physical contact,".he says. "But I want you to push them, push them hard. If they quit, that means they don't have what it takes." On the first row of bleachers rests a water cooler. Next to it sits a yellow plastic bucket. Shamrock does not like vomit left on the football field or in the bleachers.

The young men are lined up across the fifty yard line of the football field, as if for an execution squat. "Squats," barks Frank Shamrock. "Two-hundred of them. Let's go." The young men pump out the squats. They rise and fall on the infield of the football field, booming out their progress. Soon, their bodies gleam with sweat. Shamrock, wearing a tank top, shorts and tennis shoes, scans the young men with the probing eye of a casting director. "We aren't looking for big pecs and mean faces. We can build pecs and we can show a guy how to look tough," Shamrock says. "We are looking for heart." All the young men finish the squats and move to the next exercise, fifty push-ups.

On the track, a few middle-aged women have begun a brisk walk. One elbows another playfully and points out the Lion's Den fighters, their chests bared. "We've got to come out here more often, Ginger," she says.

As the push-ups continue, a young man collapses into the fescue and then struggles to rise. Bohlander is on him like a mongoose on a cobra. "Do it! You can do it! Get your butt in gear!" The mind is willing, but the young man's body trembles and shakes and finally melts into the grass. He is an earnest young man from Texas, a man who claimed he had extensive martial arts experience and seemed impressive on videotape. Shamrock walks to him. "It's over," he says. "I don't want you getting hurt. You gotta get in better shape, man." The Texan nods, rises, and staggers toward the bleachers, his legs threatening imminent collapse, his chest heaving like a bellows. He circles back after a few minutes and approaches Shamrock. "May I continue, sir? I don't like to give up." Shamrock is both firm and comforting. "You didn't give up. I told you to stop. You tried. You gave it your best. You have nothing to be ashamed of. And you can come back. You can try again. I hope you will. But for now, it's over." Resigned, the man limps to the sidelines and the role of spectator.

A piggyback carry is the next phase of torture. Each man hoists another on his back and struggles down field fifty yards. The five remaining men are weary and sweat-soaked, but they finish. They are given a minute to gulp some water, then told to scramble up the stadium steps. Bohlander and White run beside each man, watching to make sure he doesn't slip and tumble down the bleachers. The men start to drag, and they are given the verbal lashes of the proctors. "Keep moving, you fat runt," Bohlander says to one. "Don't give up. Don't give up." The five complete the stairs, but one man, well-built and burly, is suffering. He straggles down the stairs, then lumbers, like a drunk, toward the parking lot. "Hey, hey," Shamrock says, "You done?" The man doesn't answer. He just continues his groggy gait, his pride preventing the obvious reply. "Yeah," Shamrock says, to no one in particular. "I guess he's done."

There is more anguish for the dying legs: Burpees. The four who remain go to the ground, kick their legs back, bounce up, and do it again. There is no longer any effort to sound off. It is effort enough to simply remain in motion, to somehow mimic the exercise that is expected. Another, finally, collapses. He rolls over on his back and gasps. His arms are flung to each side, his eyes closed, his chest heaving, sucking oxygen into his mutinous limbs.

Three remain: Craig, Ron, and a young man named Mark. The caravan returns to the dojo. One by one, the three take turns doing chin-ups. Their bodies rise, steady at first, then twitching with exhaustion, each man desperately trying to jut his jaw over the bar. Ron finishes with thirteen, Mark with twelve, Craig with ten. Then it is to the ring. Each man faces one of the resident fighters for a series of take-downs and submissions. The men flail and flop around the ring, putting up what meager fight they can muster. But it is hopeless. The Lion's Den fighters are having a feast. Again and again, the recruits are clinched, lifted, and slammed to the canvas mat like rag dolls.

To Shamrock, it does not matter that the young men are glazed-eyed, that their limbs are enfeebled by the killing work of the last two hours, that they are barely able to defend themselves. That's expected. What matters is that they keep coming. Men with black belts have tried out and failed to make it through even the squats. "I look," Shamrock says, "for a guy who never, never, EVER gives up."

At last, the rag-doll toss is completed. The fighters are told to stand in the ring, together, to hear the verdicts. Shamrock has spoken to Bob and Frank. They've concurred. There will be nothing private about this final selection. "Two of you made it," Shamrock says. "It's Ron and Mark. And you, Craig, you have the heart. But you are too damn skinny. You'll just get thrown around. You need to get some beef on you. I hope you will come back."

The tension is broken. The fighters, those who've made it and those who haven't, exchange hugs and high-fives. Bob Shamrock passes out publicity photos of his son to those who won't be coming back.

Ken Shamrock turns to Ron and Mark. "Now. I want you to listen to me very carefully. For the next six months, I own you. Absolutely own you. Do you understand this?" The young men nod their ascent. Soon, their hair will be shaved. They will claim a bedroom or part of a bedroom in the fighters' house in the rolling farmland outside of Lodi. And they will train, train fiercely to become a modern hand-to-hand warrior.

Outside the Lion's Den, the sun is rapidly dropping, the shadows growing dark and long. Craig, the game but gangly Canadian who was not chosen, leans against the wall of the dojo, his face a mask of dejection.

"I knew I should have gained some weight," he says, rolling his eyes upwards. "I knew it."

It will be a long bus ride home.

Chapter 5

Father and Son

Susanville, California
October, 1979

T he car carrying the boy and the Napa County probation officer moves steadily through the rugged, rocky country on the eastern slope of the Sierra. The car threads its way through the town of Susanville, a settlement of 7,000 sustained largely by the jobs provided by a nearby state prison. The boy stares at the mountainous terrain and sees only isolation. "I am," thinks the boy, "going to be stuck in the middle of the boonies." The car cruises through town and, four miles outside Susanville, arrives at the driveway of a massive home. As the car moves between iron gates closer to the home, the boy rolls down the window and the scent of pines and Douglas firs floods his nostrils.

The air is crisp. A long Indian summer is ending, and soon the peaks to the west will be dusted with white. A season is changing.

The boy peers behind the imposing house and sees the rolling emerald expanse of a golf course. He sees the sky-blue of a swimming pool behind the huge house, as well, and glimpses the white-topped net of a tennis court. The car stops and the probation officer leads the boy toward the front door, a soaring entry of solid, hand-carved wood. This house, this place, is like nothing the boy had ever seen or even dreamed about.

Suddenly, the heavy door swings open. A man with bright blue eyes and a smile bounds out onto the porch and extends his hand. "Hello," he says. "I'm Bob Shamrock. Welcome to the Shamrock Ranch."

The boy was a 14-year-old incorrigible named Kenneth "Kenny" Wayne Nance. He'd been exiled from his own home for defying his parents, for fighting, and stealing. He'd spent months in the Napa County Juvenile Hall. He'd spent time in a group home where the young, rebellious boys had bullied the home operators to the point where the youths, not the adults, ruled the premises.

He'd spent time, too, in a foster home run by a police officer who wanted the boy to work like a slave on outdoor projects, while his own son lounged inside watching TV. The boy had questioned that, questioned why he should excavate a swimming pool with pick and shovel while another able-bodied young man should sit idle. The man with the badge was outraged by the boy's questions, his impudence. He erupted, locked the boy in handcuffs, ordered the thirteen-year-old taken from the home in the back of a patrol car.

And so it seemed the boy standing on the steps of the palatial Shamrock Boys Ranch on an autumn afternoon had little hope. He was a failure in school. He had no strong family ties to speak of. He was a captive in a juvenile justice system, a vast bureaucracy where many graduated to the state's Youth Authority or to state prison.

The boy said little when the man who introduced himself as Bob Shamrock shook his hand on the front porch of his mansion. The boy was quiet by nature and he'd learned to keep his mouth shut until he could size up a person or a situation, which he did quickly and well.

But the man immediately felt a connection, a powerful one. He and his wife had housed and counseled and directed more than 600 young people in this huge and meticulous home. But there was something different about this young man. His intense confidence, his dark eyes, pools of both defiance and vulnerability. There was just something about the kid. Something edgy, and something special.

Bob Shamrock had been working with troubled youngsters since 1968, when he and his wife, Dee Dee, opened a group home in Anza,

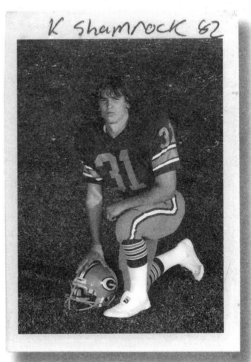

As a linebacker, Shamrock had a sixth sense for where the ball was going. He played at Lassen High School, home of the Grizzlies. *(Shamrock family photo)*

California. But Bob Shamrock had been serving and helping others all of his life. As a youngster, Shamrock assisted at a mission in downtown Los Angeles largely supported by his father, Chuck Shamrock, a devout Baptist and the owner of a prosperous testing and fabrication business. The boy served the mission as janitor, waiter, musician. "I'd go down after school and help serve up the meals. Chili or stew or bologna sandwiches," Shamrock recalled. Shamrock was also proficient on the piano, and he'd often accompany the ex-cons and winos as they belted out "The Old Rugged Cross," or "Amazing Grace." Shamrock helped out at the mission throughout his school years. He learned a sense of duty, of compassion, of service.

Occasionally the men who received nourishment and direction at the mission would ascend to lives of sobriety and success. They would drop by in suits or ties, or send notes. But Shamrock also saw the terrible fate suffered by others who lived on the street and were eventually consumed by it. "More than once my Dad and I would pull up to the mission and discover bodies in the parking lot or curled up in the mission doorway," he said. "Overdoses, many of them. It was absolutely heartbreaking."

Bob Shamrock, at a very early age, learned that he could and should make a difference in the world.

He also learned that human beings can will themselves to change, to reinvent themselves. He accomplished it himself. As a high school freshman, Shamrock was neither large nor athletic nor a stellar student. But in what he recalls as an Epiphany, he one day sensed an inner potential and an overwhelming drive to perfect it. "I did not want to be a mediocre student. I did not want a mediocre life," he said. "I resolved to do my very best, to push harder. To be somebody." So Bob Shamrock developed his natural wit, his study habits, his grades. By the time he graduated from Lynnwood High School in Southern California, Shamrock was a straight A student voted most likely to succeed. He enrolled at UCLA as a pre-med student but was eventually forced to leave his studies to help his father run the testing business.

Shamrock would not become a physician, but he would use his nimble mind and extraordinary stores of energy to help his fellow man—to make a difference—in other ways.

The Shamrocks sold their testing business in 1971. Bob and Dee Dee Shamrock had desperately wanted children yet none had graced their marriage. So they began taking young wards of the juvenile court into their home on a ranch near the town of Anza. The childless couple found caring for the young men who were runaways

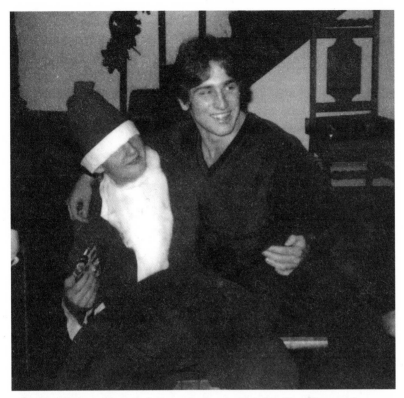

Christmas at the Shamrock home in Susanville, CA. Ken Shamrock, age 14, hams it up with one of the other boys who donned a Santa's suit. *(Shamrock family photo)*

or thieves or worse deeply satisfying. They built a reputation for running a home that was both compassionate and disciplined. A home that could make a difference in a troubled boy's life. In 1973, they founded the 6,400-square foot place on Wingfield Road in Susanville, a place with fourteen bedrooms and seven bathrooms, a place that would allow them to care for nearly twice as many young men as they had in Anza.

As Bob Shamrock stood on the porch and greeted the boy from Napa, he simply *knew.* As surely as he had known twenty-five years earlier that he could and would turn his own life around, he *knew.* This boy would be different. This boy would become the son Bob Shamrock had never had.

The Napa probation officer, his duty completed, began the journey home. The boy entered the mansion. He remained awestruck. "What," he asked himself, "am I doing here?" Some of the homes

he'd lived in were either filthy or nearly barren of furnishings. Food
was carefully rationed. Here, there were lofty ceilings and dazzling
chandeliers. There was a grand dining table of burnished wood
already set for dinner with solid pewter goblets, plates, and soup
bowls. In one corner of the dining room were soda and juice
machines. Nearby was a large bowl of fresh fruit. "You've had a long
drive," Shamrock said. "Can I get you something to drink? Some
juice or soda?"

As he sat down for an initial interview with the boy, Shamrock
already knew much about him. He knew the boy had been found
guilty of running away, of stealing, of strong-arm robbery. He learned
these things scanning the thick file sent to him by the Napa Juvenile
Probation Department. But he sensed the youth was not a hard-core
criminal. Rather, he sensed this was a boy who'd been rocked and
wounded by circumstance. There was nothing in the probation file to
indicate the boy was malicious or psychologically defective. The boy
seemed skinny but very strong for his age, one report read. Another
notation said the boy was aggressive and hot-tempered. The files also
showed the boy was street-smart, readily able to fend for and protect
himself. In common lingo, the boy was survivor.

Yet the boy did not steal unless there was a need. He was quick
to fight, the file noted, even with much larger boys, but not without
some challenge or provocation. And there was something else
Shamrock noticed, as he pored through the file, something unusual
among the young men referred to him: the boy seemed to have a clear
idea of right and wrong. The file indicated the boy had not liked the
one group home because the house parents appeared to tolerate the
youngsters smoking marijuana. The boy, according to the file, did not
abuse drugs and did not think the home parents should condone their
consumption. And the official reports recounted how the boy had
questioned why he had to work while the lawman's son did not. The
boy, according to his file, was a good worker and was quite willing to
do chores as long as he felt he was treated fairly in return. The mani-
la folder stuffed with reports and evaluations, Bob Shamrock felt,
revealed a rare personality: a raging young man, but a righteous one.

Shamrock and the boy talked over tall glasses of cola. Shamrock
told the boy about the home, how he gave much, and expected much
in return. Each of the residents was allowed to eat all the food they
liked, and it was always fresh and of the highest quality. Shamrock
also taught the young men etiquette, as each resident learned the
proper way to set a table and to proceed through a formal meal. He

taught them responsibility, as the boys all pitched in to help with cleaning, laundry, and kitchen chores and also performed community service work. The Shamrock boys split wood for widows, painted the homes of the needy or poor, even picked up trash along local roads. Shamrock offered the boys a variety of sports, including swimming, tennis, basketball, and weight lifting. Bob Shamrock loved sports himself and was often in the center of the action. "Keep them busy enough, and tired enough, and they won't get into trouble," he told friends. One of the features was an arcade room with a dozen video games on free play. And Shamrock, a car buff, owned a shiny collection that included a Camaro, a Cadillac, even a Corvette. Some of the boys, if they did well enough, were allowed the ultimate reward: they could drive one of the cars into town.

The Shamrock home was its own reward for good behavior. And the standards, in the realm of group homes, were unique. Shamrock expected his boys to work hard, play hard, pull down decent grades, and behave themselves. Yet when a kid messed up, came home late, or was caught puffing a joint, Shamrock was firm and also understanding. He talked with the youth, provided sessions with counselors, offered opportunities for redemption. "The boys," he recalled some years later, "did not come to me with angel wings attached." Many group home owners gave up on a kid after one or two foul-ups. Shamrock was more patient. He took the time to talk with his boys, understand their backgrounds, relate with them. Some boys who had bounced like pinballs among other homes spent years with Shamrock, forged life-long bonds with him. (By his own account, Shamrock's devotion to the home and the boys contributed to his divorce from Dee Dee in 1981. "I think she felt I was spending more time and effort working with the boys than working on our relationship, and she was probably right," Shamrock said.)

Shamrock preferred to take on boys who were energetic, even aggressive, to young men who were withdrawn or lethargic. He liked to keep the pace fast, the energy level high. He was also quick to spot bad blood building between his boys, and quick to stop it. The boys were invited to engage in a rough but efficient form of conflict resolution. They could put on boxing gloves and go to the backyard. There, encircled by other boys and the staff members, they would pound out their differences. Usually popcorn and sodas would be served, and the mood was more festive than vengeful. "If one boy wanted to fight and the other didn't, that was okay," Shamrock recalled. "We'd settle it with a heart-to-heart talk. But in most cases, they worked things out just fine in the backyard. Some of the guys who went at it ended up becoming pretty good friends." The boxing sessions also included boys from town who had a beef with one of the Shamrock kids. There were bruises and bloody noses suffered in such backyard fisticuffs. But order was maintained, honor upheld, poisonous feelings defused.

At first, the Nance boy from Napa felt uncomfortable in the elegant home with the huge rock fireplace and the velvet couches. But he soon learned that while the decor was formal, the house was run in a relaxed and respectful way. He found, surprisingly, that he fit in rather well. Bob Shamrock noticed the boy had a lean build and was naturally coordinated. He encouraged him to try out for sports at Lassen High School, and the boy readily agreed. With cat-like reflexes and God-given strength, he was a natural wrestler. He had a rare passion and talent for football. The boy could stick like a battering ram, but he moved with the grace and fluidity of a matador. And he had a sixth sense for where the opposition would try to strike next. "He was," Bob Shamrock said, "the most gifted athlete I had ever seen." The boy's rage did not evaporate. Instead, it was directed to the playing field and the wrestling mat. Finally, through sports, and with the encouragement of Bob Shamrock, the angry, incorrigible boy began to excel.

In his senior year, Kenny was team captain and an All-League selection at linebacker. And he was an undefeated wrestler, headed for a state championship belt, when his season ended abruptly. In practice one afternoon, Kenny hoisted another wrestler on his shoulders and prepared to drop him. Suddenly the foam-rubber wrestling mat slipped below his feet. Kenny toppled to the floor with his opponent's weight collapsing across his head and neck. There was a snap, and Kenny was rushed to the hospital with a fractured vertebrae. The surgeons screwed a metal halo into his skull to keep his spine from shifting. They told him there could be no strenuous activity for a year and no contact sports—ever again. Kenny set out to prove them wrong. Within two months, he was on the basketball court, going high on the board to pull in rebounds, the halo still embedded in his skull. The breakage, the long weeks in the halo, did nothing to slow Kenny or numb his animal drive to play, to compete, to prevail. If anything, Bob Shamrock noticed, the injury seemed to leave his charge nearly impervious to pain.

Though much of his anger was poured into sports, Kenny continued to brawl. And Bob Shamrock's instinct about the boy possessing an acute sense of right and wrong was revealed in these conflicts. When the football coach ordered players to go all-out during a practice, but leave the quarterback untouched, Kenny did not understand. It wasn't right, wasn't fair. He slipped a block, charged the quarterback, and smashed him into the turf, drawing the instant wrath of the coach. On a rainy day, when a football practice was held in the gym, the players were instructed to go half-speed. A boy who outweighed Kenny by forty pounds looking for a cheap shot threw a shoulder into Kenny, sending him sprawling to the hardwood floor. That wasn't right, wasn't fair. Kenny nailed him with a right hand, sent him down, then straddled him and pounded him bloody before the coaches could restrain him. Kenny narrowly evaded expulsion for the beating, but Bob Shamrock convinced school authorities the attack was provoked by the larger boy's cheap shot. Instead of expulsion, Kenny was suspended for five days.

When another Susanville youth defaced one of Shamrock's cars, Kenny lit into him. The incident took place at an after-game party. Kenny had been granted permission to drive one of Shamrock's cars to the party. It was a 1957 Cadillac El Dorado, a mint condition classic that was Shamrock's pride and joy. The other youth, who'd been guzzling beer, accused Kenny of trying to steal away his girlfriend. Then he smashed a beer bottle on the hood of the treasured Caddy, sending beer froth and shattered glass everywhere. Kenny struck him square on the chin with the impact of a sledgehammer and actually knocked the young man out of his shoes.

Kenny returned home and explained to Shamrock why the Caddy was coated with beer. Later that night, Shamrock was awakened by a telephone call. It was the boy Kenny had knocked shoeless. "I want to come over and put on the gloves and I want go into the backyard and finish it with Kenny," the boy said, his voice still slurred by the beer. "In your condition, that wouldn't be a very wise idea," Shamrock replied. "But if you show up, we'll get out the gloves."

A few hours later, at sunrise, Shamrock was again awakened by the phone. "I won't be coming over," the boy said. "I've sobered up, and I don't think I ever want to get hit like that again. Besides, I think my jaw may be broken."

Shamrock himself had to take on his strapping young charge one night. Under house rules, anyone using profanity was subject to having his mouth washed out with soap. Early in the evening, Kenny, acting as a peer counselor, had duly washed out the mouth of one house resident who had uttered a foul word. But an hour later,

Kenny himself had suffered a slip of the tongue. "Go wash your mouth out," Shamrock ordered. Kenny declined, and stood, cross-armed, next to the kitchen sink. Shamrock was in good shape for a man in his early forties. Still, Kenny was now close to six feet tall, weighed 180 pounds, and could bench-press 350 pounds. Shamrock grabbed a bar of soap and walked over to Kenny. "Wash your mouth," he demanded. Again, Kenny demurred. Quite unexpectedly, Shamrock kicked Kenny's feet out from under him. The boy crashed to the floor, and Shamrock dropped over him, sticking a knee on the boy's chest. He shoved the bar of soap into the boy's mouth and pushed his chin up, breaking the soap off in his mouth.

And it was over. Shamrock said the maneuver would not have been possible without divine intervention.

"I knew I couldn't back down, and I knew how strong Ken was," Shamrock said. "So I said a prayer: 'Please, God, help me take care of this.' He answered my prayer."

Kenny and Shamrock later talked about the incident, and Kenny apologized. The scuffle, in fact, only drew them closer. Kenny respect-ed Shamrock, a man who was fair but determined to dispense discipline with either his tongue or, if the need arose, with muscle. "Bob was fair. He was caring but he was not afraid to discipline me or any of the other boys," Ken said.

Kenny was gaining a reputation in Susanville and even in Reno, eighty miles to the south, as a superb athlete and a young man not to be tangled with. Shamrock was proud of the young man's athletic blos-soming. He was concerned, though, that Kenny still sometimes seemed distant and uneasy. Ken had many pals, most fellow athletes, but no close friends. "If Ken let somebody in too close, he might get hurt emo-tionally. So he kept people at a distance." The pattern was true, as well, with girlfriends. Ken would cut off a relationship before it became too deep, too emotionally intimate, too painful.

Bob Shamrock even hired a special therapist to visit the home each week and talk with Kenny, to try and explore his feelings, his emotion-al tautness. The sessions did little good. At his core, Ken remained a tightly coiled young man unable and unwilling to let anyone, even Shamrock, venture too close.

Still, while Bob Shamrock didn't entirely understand this young man, he had grown to care for him deeply. The boy had arrived at his doorstep a skinny but street-wise urchin. He was now a star athlete, a high school graduate, a young man with plans for college. While Shamrock saw the anger still sparking in the boy, he also saw the heart, the indomitable spirit that raised him high against the basket-ball backboard with a steel halo screwed into his skull. He saw a luminous future that even the boy could not.

Bob Shamrock, glib and quick-witted, had not known he was looking for a son. Still, he found one in Kenny, a young man with quiet pride and few words. Somehow, Shamrock had felt it, known it, from the start.

So in February of 1982, soon after Kenneth Wayne Nance turned eighteen, he was legally adopted by the man who had welcomed him to the Shamrock Boys Ranch on a crisp autumn day more than four years before.

From that day on, the boy would have a father, and the father a son.

From that day on, the boy would be known as Kenneth Wayne Shamrock.

Chapter 6

500 Squats

Tampa, Florida
1990

G ive me 500 squats," Sammy Saranaka barked. Ken Shamrock, stripped to a pair of shorts and tennis shoes, quickly obliged. He dropped low toward the asphalt, his powerful quadriceps tensing, then rose up explosively. "One," Shamrock sounded off. Saranaka bent down and rose, too, keeping pace with Shamrock. As a talent scout for a Japanese fighting circuit, Masami "Sammy" Saranaka had tested hundreds of aspiring warriors. Bouncers, ex-football players, pro wrestlers. There was one way to quickly check both heart and legs: squats. Most of the prospects would melt after 300. Few made it to 400. If a man could do 500 squats in the steamy afternoon heat of Tampa, Saranaka knew, he was both strong and game.

Saranaka was an agent for the Universal Wrestling Federation, based in Tokyo. It was a pro-wrestling circuit, but one whose fans thirsted for increasingly athletic performers and realistic contests. So Saranaka was not looking for 300-pound hambones. He was looking for men whose body and heart would be convincing to savvy fight fans demanding more and more fighting authenticity.

Shamrock pumped out the squats. This was no lark for him. It was serious work, important work. At age twenty-six, he had no traditional job skills to speak of, certainly nothing approaching a career. Since high school, Shamrock had dabbled and drifted. He tried many things, but none had brought him the success he dreamed of, and that his father, Bob Shamrock, felt he was destined for. The one thing he could do, do with a singular passion and power, was fight.

Yet so far, that gift had proven a bittersweet blessing.

Now a married man with a baby, Shamrock needed a break, needed it badly. Saranaka, he hoped, would give him the opportunity he desperately needed.

Following graduation from Lassen High School, Shamrock played nose guard for the football team at Shasta Community College in Redding, California. Shamrock was All-League and defensive most

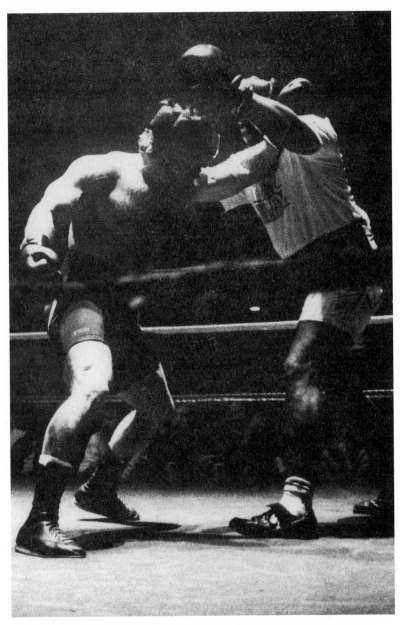

It was during his son's Toughman competitions that Bob Shamrock realized his son was a born gladiator. Shamrock won three Toughman contests, one in Redding, CA, and two in North Carolina. This fight was in 1990 in Hickory, North Carolina, where the promoters gave Shamrock the nickname "The Destroyer."
(photo by Jeff Willhelm, The Charlotte Observer)

valuable player. His tackling and tenacity were the stuff of a four-year
college football program; his grades were not.

While living in Redding, Shamrock took a job as a bouncer at a
bar called Doc's Skyroom. Though he was only nineteen, not even old
enough to sip a beer under California law, Shamrock was 210 pounds
of rapid-fire muscle, ready and able to control a boisterous barroom.
He had experience taking down bigger men through street fights and
his hyper-aggressive brand of football.

For Shamrock, bouncing was relatively easy money. He scanned
the crowd looking for the guy who was getting cocky or obnoxious.
When he found such a customer, he told him, quite politely, to cool it.
If the guy was not blitzed, Shamrock provided a drink on the house.
If the guy was already sloppy, Shamrock asked him, still very politely, but also very clearly, to leave. If the guy stared at Shamrock with
eyes glazed with beer and told Shamrock to get lost, Shamrock
advised the guy he would call the police if the guy insisted on causing a ruckus. And if the guy took a swing at Shamrock, the teen-aged
bouncer swiftly took the man down, dragged him out, and suggested
his patronage would no longer be appreciated.

Years later, Shamrock would say his work maintaining order in
barrooms taught him valuable lessons for the fighting ring: he learned
to carry himself with authority, to read body language, to remain calm
in a volatile situation.

It was in Redding that Shamrock fought in his first Toughman
contest. Such events drew bouncers, construction workers, amateur boxers, ex-football players. Guys who were tough, or thought
they were, even if they had a forty-pound gut slopping out over
their trunks. The combatants duked it out in a crude ring. The last
man standing, after fighting his way through a tournament, won
$1,000. Shamrock, fast and strong, a superb athlete, and tempered
by street fights and football, thought the Toughman would be a
sure thing. It was.

The combat was staged in a rodeo arena at the edge of town. All
of the fighters were required to wear sixteen-ounce gloves and
padded headgear. With the oversized mitts on, most of the fighters
could hit something, even if the blows carried no sting. Shamrock,
despite having his hands encased in the pillows, could sting. He
won his first bout by knockout with a single, vicious punch to his
opponent's jaw. He won his second with a flurry of body blows. He
was set to fight in the championship but the other finalist pulled out,
complaining of a broken hand. So the strapping bouncer from Doc's

Skyroom left the dusty arena that night with $1,000 and a new nick-name: Ken "One Punch" Shamrock.

In the ring during the Toughman, he would say later, Shamrock felt almost possessed. He felt so pumped, so alive, so natural. He had been electrified and driven by the rage. In both bouts, he had moved relentlessly forward, throwing punch after punch after punch. His Dad, Bob Shamrock, had coached and cheered from ringside. Watching his son so quickly and deftly destroy other men, he was convinced. "I knew," he recalled, "that Ken was a natural gladiator."

Yet there were few help wanted ads for gladiators. So after two years playing football at Shasta, and no real prospects for a four-year college, Shamrock's best option appeared to be the military. He signed up with the U.S. Marines. He flourished in the disciplined, competitive, and highly physical atmosphere of Camp Pendleton. He was selected as a platoon leader. "Some recruits despised boot camp. I actually liked it," he said. But military physicians conducting a routine examination discovered the old vertebrae injury from high school. Grudgingly, Marine officials discharged Shamrock from boot camp after six weeks. Though his career as a leatherneck was short-lived, Shamrock learned a critical lesson, one he would apply in coming years: to survive in a war, you must be prepared. You must train and prepare as part of a close-knit group. You must know yourself, your weapons, your enemy.

A career in the Marines, like the vision of a four-year college, had proven evasive. Shamrock moved to Reno and again found work as a bouncer, this time at a popular night spot called the Premiere Club. He also began to moonlight as a male dancer. Though quiet, Shamrock, dark and handsome and well-muscled, was popular among the female customers of the club. One night, when a male dance revue performed, the crowd of women began a chant: "Ken-nee! Ken-nee! Ken-nee!" Shamrock obliged, the performance was wildly received, and for a couple of years he earned pin money by performing in clubs, at private parties, and even at the Nevada governor's mansion for a fund-raiser sponsored by Republicans. At the political event Shamrock and his friend and fellow bouncer and dancer, Remi Bruyninga, posed for individual photos with bejeweled Republican wives. "We were like bookends," Bruyninga said. "Kenny on one side and me on the other." The men wore nothing but cuffs, collars, black tights, and broad smiles. Shamrock, according to Bruyninga, showed a surprising ease whenever he was on stage. "Kenny is not a big talker. But get him in front of a crowd, and he is a natural performer," he said. The quality would be revealed time and time again in future years. When he entered a room, people would turn and notice. He was a man of relatively few words, and would remain so. But when he spoke, people listened. Shamrock, in the phrasing of entertainment and politics, possessed an undeniable charisma.

In Reno, Shamrock's reputation as a fighter and a dangerous bad-ass continued to grow. Shamrock liked to prowl after-hour parties. Sometimes he was accompanied by his pal Bruyninga. And sometimes the two men, both muscular and self-confident, would rumble. "We were at a bar late one night and some guys started giving me a hard time," Bruyninga called. "I just tried to stay calm. When I got up to go use the rest room, I told Kenny, 'look, don't do anything while I'm gone.' I come back from the rest room and five guys are sleeping on the floor, courtesy of Kenny. I said, 'man, I thought you weren't going to do any-thing.' He told me he couldn't help it, they jumped him."

It was in the early morning hours of July 19, 1987 that Shamrock hurt a man.

At twenty-two, the Reno man was tall, strong, athletic, and trou-bled. He had been an All-State football player at a high school in the Reno area. His size and uncanny speed attracted a slew of college scouts. The young man chose Brigham Young University in Provo, Utah, becoming the school's first blue-chip football recruit. As a sophomore tight end, he was selected as a third-string All-American. His life beyond the gridiron, though, was not so auspicious. A non-Mormon, the young man, according to the *Reno Gazette-Journal* news-paper, was frequently reprimanded by college authorities for violation of the school's strict code of honor. The code, among other provisions, forbade the consumption of alcohol.

As a freshman, the young man began using Percodan, a painkiller. After suffering a fracture of his foot, his use of the drug increased. Ultimately, he became addicted to the pills. The young Reno man and two other players were charged with forging prescrip-tions for Percodan and they were admitted to an in-patient drug reha-bilitation center in Utah. The players held a news conference after their release describing the dangers of drug abuse. "It brought me," the young man said, "to my knees." Four months later, however, he was again convicted of prescription drug charges. This time, he was sentenced to ten days in jail and a $500 fine. And this time, he was expelled from Brigham Young University.

So on that summer night at the Premiere Club, the Reno man had a clouded future. He began drinking, and according to Shamrock and

Bruyninga, he drank too much. "I was in the middle of it," Bruyninga said. "We tossed the guy out because he got in a scuffle with another customer. He wanted to get back in. 'Just go home,' I told him. He didn't want to go home. He kept pointing at Shamrock and saying 'I want a piece of him.' I told him, 'no, believe me, dude, you do not want a piece of that man.' But I finally couldn't hold him back anymore. 'You want him, you go ahead,' I said. He charged and Kenny hit him. The guy went down and he didn't get up. He was messed up."

The young man, in fact, was rushed to the hospital with a massive blood clot in his brain. He underwent extensive surgery at the Washoe Medical Center during which a piece of his skull was removed.

The young man later told a reporter for the Gazette-Journal that he was lucky to survive his confrontation with Shamrock. The blood clot that had been surgically pulled from his head, he said, was the size of a grapefruit.

Reno police, according to a department spokesman, found differing versions of what had happened in the early morning hours of July 19 at the Premiere Club. They ruled the case "mutual combat." The District Attorney declined to press charges against Shamrock or the former football player.

Even so, the young man later sued the Premiere Club and Shamrock. The Premiere, soon after the lawsuit was filed, moved for bankruptcy court protection. At the end of 1996, the case had still not been fully resolved. Bruyninga feels the young man himself was responsible for his injuries. "It was his own doing," he said. "When he ran into Kenny, he ran into the wrong man."

A few weeks after the incident, before the Premiere had closed, a tall, striking young woman entered the club. Her name was Tina Ramirez. She had beautiful black hair and eyes of shimmering green and gold. Ramirez, originally from San Diego, was working as an airlines reservation supervisor in Reno. As part of a ladies' night promotion, Shamrock was pouring free champagne and handing out roses to all female patrons. "He had long hair and a mustache and love handles," Ramirez said. "But you could tell he had a good build. He had a nice chest." Ramirez, with a bright and buoyant personality, took a few sips of champagne and ventured over to the man with the nice chest. "Would you like to dance?," she offered. He did.

And so began a friendship that would bloom into marriage for Tina Ramirez and Ken Shamrock. In the first few weeks of their courtship, Ramirez was puzzled by her friend's reticence. "He didn't seem to have anything to say," she recalled. "In fact, I was ready to call it quits. I just thought he was rather boring. I thought maybe he was just a dumb jock." But on what may have been the couple's final meeting, a dinner in the apartment where Ramirez was living, Shamrock started opening up. "He seemed more comfortable, more relaxed. He just started talking, and the things he was saying made sense. He didn't seem boring at all. He was interesting. Pretty soon, we became best friends." She found there was more to like about the man than just a well-developed chest. She found him an intriguing blend of macho and innocence. "I could almost look through him and see a little boy deep inside," she said. "He seemed vulnerable." She was also impressed with his gentlemanly etiquette, the result of his upbringing in the rough-but-mannered Shamrock ranch for boys. "Ken always opened the car door for me. Always," she said. "I found out later he had forgotten to open the car for his date on prom night, and his dad had threatened to punch him in the stomach for it. He never forgot that."

But along with the courtesy and boyishness, she witnessed Shamrock's ferocity, and it nearly drove her away. The couple, engaged to wed, attended a New Year's Eve party together with friends in Reno. A man who had imbibed too much growled raunchy comments toward one of the women in the Shamrock party. Shamrock instantly shot to his feet. "Ken told the guy to watch his mouth," Ramirez recalled. "And the guy didn't back off or shut up. Ken got right up close to the guy and he pushed Ken. After that, it was a blur. Ken's hand came up very fast and, boom, the man went down very fast." As was typical, Shamrock had not started the fight, but he had not avoided it, either. Tina Ramirez was fuming. Here was the man who would be her husband, the future father of her children, and he was inviting trouble with his hair-trigger fists. "I said if he wanted to get married and have a family, he had to learn to walk away from a fight," she said. Shamrock, though, said little. His eyes were still ignited and focused like the eyes of a raptor seizing prey. It was not the last time Tina Ramirez would see this in the eyes of the man she loved. For Shamrock, the instinct to fight, fueled by a deep-seated rage, would prove difficult to extinguish.

Despite Shamrock's eruption, the engagement survived, and the couple was married on May 21, 1988 in Chula Vista, California. It was, in fact, an inspired blend of personalities: Tina a strong and verbal woman with a sparkling sense of humor, Ken a proud and plainspoken man of deceptive complexity.

Following the wedding and marriage, the couple returned to

Reno, where Shamrock took a job as a youth counselor at the Rite of Passage boys' ranch at a remote site near Yerington, Nevada. On weekends, he worked painting houses.

Though he had not wrestled consistently since high school, Shamrock decided to enter 'the Olympic heavyweight freestyle wrestling trials being held in Reno in the spring of 1988. He did surprisingly well, beating his first two opponents before losing on points. Though Shamrock's Olympic quest was inspired, like the shot at college, like the shot at the Marines, it seemed yet another lesson in futility.

Bob Shamrock remained convinced his son would someday do more than apply paint and toil at a youth camp. He persuaded Shamrock to visit a pro-wrestling school in Sacramento, California. Shamrock tried out and did well at the Buzz Sawyer Wrestling Academy, well enough to be accepted. So for several months, father and son made the six-hour round trip to Sacramento so the younger Shamrock could learn the lifts and throws and rolls of the professional wrestling game. In late 1988, Bob Shamrock learned of another school, this one in North Carolina, a school that might spring his son directly into the world of pro-wrestling.

Bob Shamrock gave up the group home to help shepherd his son's embryonic pro-wrestling career. He made the move to Mooresville, North Carolina, along with Ken and Tina, and one other Shamrock. The young couple now had a son, Ryan Robert Shamrock, born November 24, 1988 in St. Mary's Hospital in Reno.

Shamrock had wanted badly to become a father. His dream, he shared with Tina before they were married, was to create a large family far different from his own: intact, happy, loving. Now, with the arrival of Ryan, a happy baby with dark, shiny eyes, the dream was coming true. Shamrock pampered the boy, frequently holding the infant in his massive arms and feeding him from a bottle. He also bought a baby pack and proudly carried baby Ryan across his stomach.

The new father was a hit at Nelson Royal's wrestling school in Mooresville. As the elder Shamrock suspected, the school did prove a springboard to professional work. After a few months of training, Shamrock became "Vinnie Torrelli," also known as "Mr. Wrestling." Shamrock and other wrestlers toured the small and mid-sized cities in the Southeast, usually putting on shows in National Guard armories. Shamrock was adept at the faint and flourish of pro-wrestling. "There were a few times he went down and I thought he was actually hurt," Bob Shamrock said. "But it was all part of the show."

The pay was far from princely, so Shamrock took whatever side jobs came his way. He did a stint as a bodyguard for Michael Jordan during one of the basketball star's trips to North Carolina. He also fought. Some of the contests were back-alley affairs called "squats" where two fighters would face off inside a ring of spectators, most with cash riding on the outcome. "I remember one night I got a call from a friend who said he had a squat all lined up for me. He showed up about twenty minutes later with a stumpy little dude. The dude looked at me and said 'I can take him.' So we walked out to the front yard. I pop this guy a good one in the mouth and he goes down. He wipes the blood off, jumps up, and just starts running into the night. He never looked back and never slowed down. Just disappeared in the darkness." That skirmish, though, was just a preliminary event. Shamrock and his friend proceeded to a bar on the edge of Mooresville, where a huge man with long, greasy blonde hair was waiting. Shamrock and the big blonde stepped into the parking lot behind the bar, into a ring of men. To one side was a Chevy pick-up truck with a pile of cash on the hood. The fight began and Shamrock smashed the man between the eyes, sending him sprawling to the pavement. "I asked the guy if he'd had enough. I didn't want to get injured and I didn't want to injure anybody else if I could help it. And the guy said, 'bull. This is going to be a long night for you, you son-of-a-bitch.' He's crumpled in a heap on the ground, wiping blood from his eyes, and he's threatening me. He staggered to his feet and I suplexed him, grabbed him and raised him and dropped him on his head. I asked him again if he'd had enough. 'Yeah, you son-of-a-bitch. That's enough,' he said." Shamrock went home unscathed to his sleeping wife and baby with $350 cash in his pocket; $50 from the split-second fight in the front yard and $300 from the rapid annihilation of the big man with the greasy hair.

Shamrock also fought and won two more Toughman contests while in North Carolina. One, held in Hickory in January 1990, drew a crowd of 3,000 and a reporter from the Charlotte Observer. "At 225 pounds, Ken 'The Destroyer' Shamrock of Mooresville looked like a vision of death, from his black boxing shoes and trunks to his muscle-bound shoulders," he wrote. The scribe duly noted that Shamrock won the heavyweight division and $1,000 by pummeling Scott Curtis of Granite Falls. Bob Shamrock, who rushed to congratulate his son after the final fight, noticed something, as well: his son seemed unable to see or hear him. "He was so excited up, so focused. He continued staring at the ring, staring at his opponent." Tina Shamrock witnessed the same thing. "It was like he was still in the ring. Bob was trying to talk to him, and he didn't hear him. He was like in a trance. It was kind of scary." It reminded her of the night in Reno, when his eyes remained bright and angry for long minutes after the fight. Like his father, Shamrock's wife now realized he was different. He had rare mettle and heart and an intensity, when confronted, that was absolutely frightening.

Yet there was another fight in North Carolina that Shamrock did not win, could not win, this against some of his fellow pro wrestlers.

In the world of pro-wrestling a gimmick is the act or persona a wrestler takes on, be it mountain man or cowboy or psycho. According to several people who know them, there is a tag-team that is crude and abusive in the ring and out. Their gimmick, some feel, is not unlike the way they are in real life.

In 1990, at a club in Charlotte, several pro wrestlers, including Shamrock and the members of the tag-team, were enjoying drinks. According to Shamrock, the tag-team wrestlers started hassling another wrestler, a smaller man who was with his girlfriend. When one member of the tag-team started disrespecting the woman, Shamrock told him to back off. The wrestler refused, and tried to shove Shamrock. A bouncer interceded and convinced Shamrock to relax. "They're assholes, Ken. They aren't worth it," he told Shamrock. Shamrock agreed and left for another part of the club. Later in the evening, though, he was told the taunting and disrespect had resumed after he had moved away. Infuriated, and with a few drinks under his belt, Shamrock returned to the hotel where the wrestlers were all staying. He went to the wrestlers' room and demanded they let him in. The door opened and Shamrock entered. He saw one of the men, apparently passed out, on a bed. And then he felt it, suddenly, a jarring blow to the back of the head.

When Tina Shamrock walked into the hospital room, she did not recognize her husband. He was flat on his back. His face was grotesquely swollen, both eyes purple and bloated shut. His nose was broken. His cheekbone was cracked. He had suffered broken ribs and a broken sternum, a concussion and internal injuries. Before she entered the hospital room, Tina Shamrock had been warned by the doctor of her patient's gruesome condition. He added that the injuries may have been life-threatening to a man who was not in the extraordinary physical condition of her husband.

Though her husband could not speak, Tina Shamrock knew the injuries were the result of some kind of confrontation. Despite her husband's pitiful situation, she issued a scornful tongue-lashing.

You are thoughtless and irresponsible, she said.

You very nearly left your wife without a husband, she said.

You very nearly left your son without a father, she said.

If you truly love your family, she said, you will stop fighting, you will learn, finally learn, to walk away from a fight.

Shamrock could not respond. But he heard the words. He knew his wife was right. If he wanted to be a good father, to raise the large and happy family he dreamed of, he would have to change. He would have to subdue the rage.

After his release from Charlotte Memorial Hospital, Ken Shamrock was driven home by his father. Tina Shamrock was also in the car. As the car passed a Baptist church, the church's bulletin board caught Tina Shamrock's eye. She nudged her husband and insisted he read the message, too: "A Fool Is One Who Does Not Learn From His Mistakes." Shamrock nodded and smiled.

To their credit, the wrestlers later stopped by the Shamrock house. They were not pointedly apologetic, however, nor was Shamrock especially forgiving. "I will not be pressing charges," he told them. "But you guys have one coming." There have been few words spoken among the men since. After a period of recuperation and rehab, Shamrock heard of a new opportunity. One of his friends, Dean Malenko, also a pro wrestler, said there was a place in Tampa where Shamrock could try out for a fighting circuit in Japan. The action was more realistic and the money could be very good, Shamrock learned. The idea appealed to him. Though he was perfectly adept at the burlesque of pro-wrestling, he was an athlete with legitimate credentials and aspirations. He did not want to be drifting around National Guard armories as "Vinnie Torrelli" any longer than necessary. So in 1991, he flew to Tampa and the appointment with Sammy Saranaka.

The Florida sun and humidity had drained Saranaka. He couldn't keep up. After 300 squats and moved to the shade. But Shamrock continued with the squats. He dropped down and exploded up one last time. "That's 500," he said. Saranaka said nothing, but he was pleased. The man was strong, he now knew. Exceptionally strong. "Inside," he motioned to Shamrock. "Inside we continue test." Shamrock followed the wiry talent scout into a combination dojo and gym. In the center was a fighting ring. "Get in there," Saranaka told Shamrock. He obeyed. Two men were sparring in a corner of the building and Saranaka called one of them over. "Get in there," he told the man. "You two fight." Shamrock and the other man grappled for perhaps five minutes, with Shamrock dominating. "Okay," Saranaka said. "Now a tougher fight." He called another man into the ring to face Shamrock and Shamrock again dominated. Saranaka was still silent but he was increasingly impressed. Few recruits passed the squat test. Those who did had little strength left to fight. This man was still standing, still game. But Saranaka had one more fighter to throw at this fast and tenacious prospect. "We do one more time," Saranaka told Shamrock. He called a third and final fighter to the ring. The third fighter entered the ring and began grappling with Shamrock. The fighter was small and quick so Shamrock tried to use his superior strength to wear him down. It was a tougher test, but again Shamrock prevailed. He returned to Mooresville and awaited word from Saranaka. He liked the straightforward talent scout. He was eager for a new chance with a new group in a new country. Finally, the call came. And Shamrock heard the words he'd hoped for from Masami "Sammy" Saranaka.

"Pack for Japan."

Chapter 7

America's Most Dangerous

Lodi
April 2, 1996

D id you hear? They thought Severn had a heart attack last weekend." Shamrock, his wife, Tina, and his dad, Bob, are at Coco's, one of their favorite restaurants in Lodi. Shamrock is devouring a platter of pasta and chicken along with garlic toast and salad, a fruit bowl, and tortilla soup. It's a light lunch.

A friend has joined them, and passed along word of Severn's apparent ill health. Shamrock's face grows taut with concern. "No. I had no idea. Is he okay?," Shamrock replies. "Oh, he's fine. They found it wasn't a heart attack, after all," the friend says. "They did tests and found there was no way Severn could finish a heart attack." The group breaks into relieved laughter.

Dan Severn, though a daunting opponent, also carries a stigma: he cannot finish a fight. He can clumsily pound away at an opponent with his bowling-ball sized fists. He can grind them with his bulk and brute strength. Yet he lacks the finishing chokes and holds, so central to Shamrock's submission fighting system, that allow a fighter to finish a contest decisively.

Shamrock, in fact, seems relatively unworried about the upcoming rematch with Severn. "I don't think it will be that different from the first fight," he says, planting his fork into a chunk of chicken breast. "He'll be coming at me. I'll finish him with a choke or a submission."

The Shamrocks on this day are in a light mood, and for good reason. Ken Shamrock is the budding superstar of a sport that has quickly drawn the public's fascination. He is being asked to appear in his own series of training videos and in a line of comic books. He is being wooed to endorse a line of fitness equipment. He has offers to fight in Tokyo, in Moscow, in Rio De Janeiro.

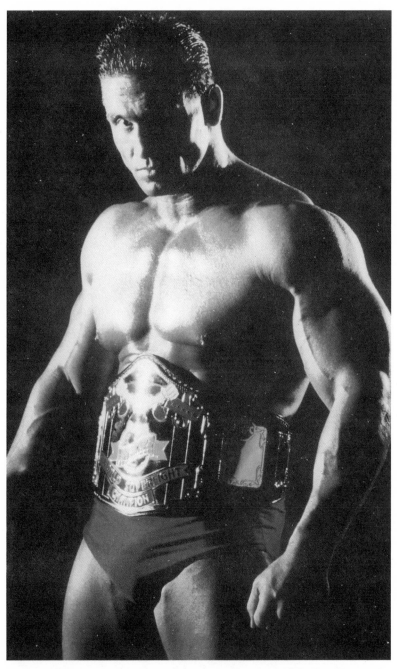

In early 1996, as the first Superfight champion of the UFC, Ken Shamrock was the most feared, and sought-after, martial artist in the country. *(Lion's Den photo)*

And they want him to make movies. Shamrock had a short, non-speaking role in *Virtuosity*, starring Denzel Washington. Shamrock played, fittingly enough, a fighter in a UFC-style combat ring. It was a small role, but Shamrock, with a physique that would put Van Damme to shame and a face reminiscent of Robert DeNiro, impressed. He landed a more substantial role in a movie titled *Champions*, backed by real estate developer Jay Wilton of Beverly Hills. Wilton is an avid weight lifter, a self-made millionaire, and former football player at Boston University. He was drawn to the physical courage of those who compete in no-holds-barred contests liked the UFC. He felt one of the fighters might be right for a featured role in *Champions*, which he financed. On a hunch, Wilton sought out Shamrock. The two spent much of a day together in Los Angeles, lifting weights, sharing lunch, and talking about life, family, and work. Wilton ended up convinced Shamrock would be perfect for his movie.

"I see Ken as a hero, as a modern-day warrior, willing to put it all one the line," he said. "After spending time with him, I felt he has true charisma, charisma I felt could be translated to the big screen."

So these days Shamrock is shuttling between Hollywood, where *Champions* is being shot, and Lodi, where he is training. The shooting schedule, Shamrock concedes, has compromised his preparation for Severn. "I knew when I took the role that I would not be able to train the way I want to train. But the film, and acting in general, represents an opportunity for my family and my future that I can't pass up," he says.

While fighting for Pancrase and the UFC has provided Shamrock with a comfortable living, acting could be even more lucrative. Several martial artists, none with Shamrock's credentials in reality fighting, have become movie stars. Featured roles in even grade B movies can pay $50,000 or more. A good role in a major production could bring Shamrock a paycheck well into six figures. "Acting is repetition. You have to do a scene time and time again," Shamrock said. "That's the tough part. But the acting itself, projecting yourself into a certain role, I find comes pretty naturally." Shamrock's hope is to become an action film star whose work transcends fight scenes.

Shamrock has emerged as the closest thing freestyle fighting has to a media darling.

On the preceding weekend, Shamrock was featured in a CBS special called "America's Most Dangerous." Along with a profile on Shamrock, the program included a look at lethal injections, killer mushrooms, and convenience store clerks who are shot on the job.

Told in advance of the show's fascination with things either dangerous or downright deadly, Tina Shamrock quipped: "I'm surprised I've survived so long." Shamrock was featured in the final segment, which began with a teaser more fitting for a war criminal than an champion martial artist. "Most of us believe in the philosophy of live and let live. *Most* of us," intoned narrator Stacy Keach. "Unfortunately, some human beings are capable of anything. They are the world's most dangerous people." Despite the ominous introduction, the piece was generally positive, tracing Shamrock's career as a reality fighting champion and highlighting his role as a husband and father.

In the final scene, Shamrock talked about the ethics of life, and of fighting. "With sports, if you break the rules, you have to pay a price. And it's the same in life," Shamrock said, looking directly into the camera. "If you break the rules, you must pay a price and those around you pay also. That's your team, or your family."

Shamrock's own family has grown steadily since the birth of son Ryan in Reno eight years ago. Ken and Tina Shamrock have been blessed with two more sons: Connor, born in 1991 in San Diego, and Sean, born in 1993 in Lodi. And Tina is pregnant with their fourth child.

Shamrock knows he must move aggressively now to provide for coming years, years when his body will not allow him to easily subdue other men with his bare hands. Those who employ Shamrock and other fighters typically do not provide pensions or 401K plans. They do not provide long-term health insurance. A fighter's success, financial and otherwise, can be all too fleeting. A study compiled by a sociologist in the 1950s provided a grim look at the occupational progression of boxing champs and leading contenders. Most were either bartenders, fight trainers, or unskilled laborers. There was a smattering of news vendors and gas station attendants.

Shamrock has no desire to be pumping gas at age sixty-five. He is painfully aware that, in terms of building a financial foundation, the future is now.

He and Tina, in fact, are hoping to purchase a ranch in the rolling hills outside of Lodi, near the town of Clements. The spread is dappled by Valley oaks and includes a comfortable main ranch house, plenty big enough for the growing Shamrock brood. There is space to build a new Lion's Den training center and living quarters for the fighters. The couple hope Bob, now running a group home for boys in nearby Lockeford, and Tina's parents, Robert and Yolanda Ramirez, will also live on the property. The ranch is in escrow and

loan officers, not accustomed to providing mortgage capital to professional hand-to-hand fighters, are cautiously combing through the
loan application.

The ranch would be another piece of Shamrock's dream. The
dream of an extended but close-knit family. Secure. Caring. Content.
The man who had no stable family life as a child himself is commit-
ted to providing a good and wholesome life for his own children.

Yet for Shamrock, being a family man has been no simple task.
There have been the trials of travel and the stresses of competition.
There have been, too, the lasting scars of a nightmarish childhood.
Part of him remains closed off, sealed. There are times, in fact, when
Shamrock has disappeared for a day or even two, pulling away, com-
municating with no one.

Shamrock's father and wife and children have shown him how to
love. But there is still a part of his soul that no one can touch.

It is only in the last few years that Shamrock has been able to com-
municate more openly with his wife and children. To do what for much
of his life he could not: express his feelings without fear of being reject-
ed or ridiculed.

So, with little in his own early childhood to guide him, Shamrock
struggles to be a loving father. The boys all attend a private Christian
school in Lodi and on the mornings when he is in town, Shamrock
drops his boys off at school. He spends as much time as he can with
his sons, attending school and sports events, and he serves as a volunteer coach for Ryan's T-ball team.

Tina was once nervous about how her husband would discipline
their sons, each spirited and energetic. While she does not oppose
spanking, she was afraid her husband, so strong and still quick-tem-
pered at times, might be too rough, too severe. He has proven to be a
stern father, she says, but a sensitive one. "Last night, he warned
Sean to finish his dinner or he would have to go to bed. Sean refused
to eat, so Ken ordered him to bed. But after a few minutes, Ken went
down to Sean's room and sat on the bed next to him. He was there for
a long time, just talking to Sean, explaining to him why it was important to follow directions and why he had to send him to his room."

Ken Shamrock, a natural-born warrior, has learned to change dia-
pers, to rise in the middle of the night to check on a sick child, to discipline with restraint. It is what Shamrock has overcome, not merely
what he has achieved, that impresses so many. Wilton, the developer
and Hollywood producer, was struck by Shamrock's decency as much
as his charisma. "Given his abusive childhood, he has all the things he

should not: a great career, a wonderful family, a tremendous set of personal principles," Wilton said. "He has sought out and created a strong family for himself; I see that as the ultimate statement of manhood."

Shamrock has finished his chicken and salad and soup. He glances at his watch and his eyes flicker with panic. "Oh, man," he says. Shamrock hastily wipes his lips with a napkin and slides out of the booth. "I gotta get going."

America's most dangerous man, it seems, is late for T-ball practice.

Chapter 8

Roll of the Dice

Manhattan
July 1993

Robert Meyrowitz played with the questions again and again as he looked out from his office perched high above East 57th Street in Manhattan. If you had a freestyle martial arts tournament and anybody could enter, Meyrowitz wondered, who would win? Which is the most efficient martial arts style? And above all, this: among the millions of martial artists on the globe, who is the best?

The questions had intrigued the entertainment executive since the day he had finally confronted his friend, the one who practiced taekwondo and constantly boasted of its benefits. "Okay," Meyrowitz said. "If taekwondo is so tough, could you take a karate guy?" "It doesn't work that way," the friend said. "They are totally different arts." "What do you mean? If you got in there with a karate guy, who would win? You or the karate guy? It's a simple question," Meyrowitz said. His friend grew flustered. "Bob, you don't get it. You don't fight people from other martial arts. It doesn't happen."

But maybe it should, Meyrowitz thought to himself. Maybe it should.

The owner of Semaphore Entertainment Group, Meyrowitz is a dapper man with a penchant for polo and imported cigars. And risk-taking. He had originally planned to be a lawyer, had even been accepted at Brooklyn Law School after earning a bachelor's degree in history at Syracuse University. But the law, for Meyrowitz, did not seem bold enough, adventurous enough. So he went into entertainment, starting as an underling at a television network and eventually rising to create and oversee his own shows. At fifty, he had produced more HBO comedy and music specials than anyone. He was, however, becoming somewhat bored with it. No matter how popular his shows were, the money remained at the flat amount agreed to by Meyrowitz and the cable giant. In recent years he'd found a new arena, one he felt offered huge new possibilities: Pay-per-view television. A potential money machine with more than twenty-five million

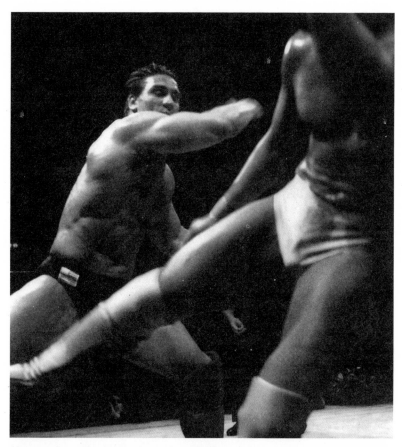

Shamrock, a star in the Pancrase fighting circuit in Japan, felt confident he would be the victor in the Ultimate Fighting Championship in Denver. Here, Shamrock swings at Pancrase fighter Takahashi in a fight in Tokyo. (photo by M. Gigie, Pancrase Hybrid Wrestling)

households around the world connected to it. Find the right show, the right button, and those households, at least enough to make it worthwhile, would kick out $10 or $20 or even $30. Clearly, you did not need all twenty-five million households to make it work. Just a fraction, even half of one percent, and the money would come gushing in.

"Pay-per-view is basically a roll of the dice," he said a few years later. "The stakes are huge. You can lose big and you can win big." Meyrowitz scored very big with a concert featuring a band of teeny-bopper heartthrobs called The New Kids on The Block. The concert became the most profitable pay-per-view entertainment event in history. But the key was not just finding the hot button on the global money machine. It was keeping costs low. Meyrowitz knew he could stage a concert with, say, the Rolling Stones, and draw a huge audience. But the guarantee he would pay for a band such as The Stones would gobble up his profits. Meyrowitz had booked The New Kids several months before their popularity really ignited. So with a blend of luck and savvy, he had invested a moderate amount, and the pay-per-view money machine had produced a jackpot.

Now he was looking for a new challenge, a new button to push. In the days after his conversation with the friend studying taekwondo, he began thinking about a radical event: a confluence of gladiators who would compete in a televised, no-holds-barred tournament. It would be real. It would be a wickedly entertaining, perhaps bloody. Definitely controversial. It would, thought Robert Meyrowitz, be the ultimate fight.

As it turned out, his instinct was right. People would pay good money to watch a freestyle fighting tournament featuring martial artists. Very good money. But it was not a karate guy or a taekwondo guy who would win the first Ultimate Fighting Championship, as it was dubbed. The first UFC, held in Denver, Colorado, was an adrenaline rush of surprises. In less than two hours, the UFC pushed contemporary martial arts back to its fight-to-survive beginnings. And it introduced a pair of extraordinary fighters, one named Gracie who had learned his art in Brazil, the other named Shamrock who had polished his technique in Japan.

At the time Meyrowitz was refining his concept in Manhattan,

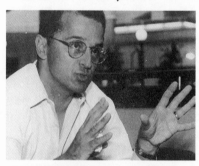

As a U.S. Marine on R and R in Bangkok, Art Davie witnesses a mixed martial arts match that eventually helped inspire the Ultimate Fighting Championship. (Calixtro Romias photo)

Art Davie was on the other edge of the continent, in Los Angeles, preparing to stage just such an event with the help of some friends. Davie is a glib adman, a former U.S. Marine, and Golden Gloves boxer. He had seen just one mixed-martial arts battle but he had never forgotten it. In 1969, he was a young Marine on R and R in Bangkok, Thailand. In a smoky saloon that doubled as a fight arena, Davie witnessed an East Indian wrestler take on a muay

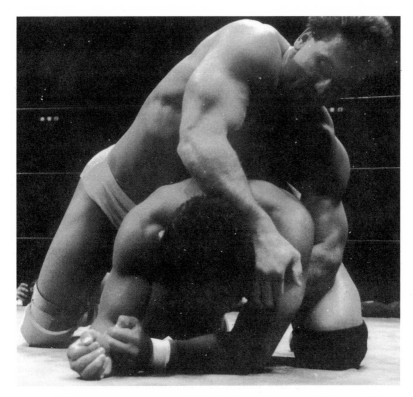

Shamrock quickly became one of the dominant Pancrase fighters, claiming victories against all of the top Pancrase competitors, including Suzuki, here trying to fend off Shamrock's attempts at an armbar or rear choke. (photo by M. Gigie, Pancrase Hybrid Wrestling)

Thai kickboxer. After a few minutes, the kickboxer finished the fight with a knee to the wrestler's head. The fight was very swift, the interplay of technique subtle and fascinating. And the fight was flat-out exciting, with no one knowing how the collision of styles would go. As his career in advertising and promotions climbed, Davie remained captivated by the idea of mixed tournaments where fighters of every discipline were welcome, where no holds were barred. Where anything could happen.

Now, in the summer of 1993, he was organizing just such a competition.

Searching for a fighter to be featured in a promotion for Tecate beer, his wanderings had taken him to Torrance, a Los Angeles suburb, to a man named Rorian Gracie. Gracie, handsome and ambitious, had trained Mel Gibson for action scenes in *Lethal Weapon* and

Lethal Weapon III. Gracie's family, originally from Brazil, practiced their brand of ju-jitsu at a popular academy. In Brazil, the Gracies boasted a long history of taking on and beating all comers in any-thing-goes matches. Eager to showcase his family's fighting prowess, Rorian Gracie agreed with Davie that the timing was perfect for a wide-open tournament—one he was convinced would be won by a Gracie. There was a student at the academy who might add just the right creative power to such a production: John Milius, a Hollywood director, producer, and writer with numerous major film credits, including *Apocalypse Now* and *Conan the Barbarian*.

Davie and Gracie could line up the fighters. Milius could add a stylish theatrical touch. But they needed someone who could pack-age the event, market it, and feed it to the global pay-per-view money machine. They contacted a small but innovative company in Manhattan, one that had pioneered pay-per-view programs. There, they enjoyed a surprisingly receptive audience from the president of the company, a man named Robert Meyrowitz.

Within weeks of the initial discussions, a radical pay-per-view sports event was being hawked to cable television stations across the country; men from the far reaches of the Earth would converge and battle in a bare-knuckle tournament for a grand prize of $50,000.

Ken Shamrock was confident the purse would be his. He had traveled far from his days of swift knock-outs in alleys and rodeo are-nas. After the successful try-out with Sammy Saranaka in Tampa, Shamrock had fought and flourished in Japan. He had begun with a grueling try-out in the dojo of the Universal Wrestling Federation on the outskirts of Tokyo.

The beginners, the young boys, actually lived in the dojo, cook-ing and cleaning for the veteran fighters. For the try-out, Shamrock was first matched against a young boy. The two sparred ferociously for twenty minutes, neither gaining an advantage. Shamrock was far stronger, but the compact Japanese fighter was quick and skilled. Shamrock faced another young boy for twenty minutes more and again he held his own. But then Shamrock faced Suzuki, one of the best of the Japanese fighters, and he was humiliated. Suzuki submitted him with a kneebar, a lock that puts tendon-popping pressure on the joint. Tiring, stunned by the pain of the kneebar, Shamrock then faced Funaki, perhaps the finest of the Japanese fighters. Funaki quickly choked Shamrock, then placed him in an ankle lock, then submitted him with an armbar.

It was sixty minutes of hell. Shamrock was beaten and dazed and embarrassed. He rolled against a wall and sat, sweating and trying to catch his breath. It was wrong, he thought. This was all wrong. It would never work. He was not able to keep up with the quicker, more skilled Japanese. For Shamrock, a dull panic set in. He was a husband and father, a man approaching thirty. Yet he had no job skills to speak of. He had worked intermittently as a youth counselor, a painter, a bouncer, a professional wrestler. He had been released from the Marine Corps because of an old wrestling injury. He had hoped, desperately, that Japan would be a land of new opportunity.

Where would he go now?

Then Funaki, one of the fighters who spoke good English, came over and stood in front of him. Shamrock expected a terse rejection, an order to collect his belongings and return home. It did not come.

"Did good," Funaki said. "Did not give up."

Shamrock, suddenly elated, wobbled to his feet and shook Funaki's hand. "You stay here in Japan," Funaki said. "You learn to fight with us."

And so Ken Shamrock was accepted, at the age of twenty-seven, as an apprentice fighter, a young boy. Shamrock stayed in Japan for two months, eating heaping bowls of rice and teriyaki chicken and fish and fetching towels for sweaty veterans. Mainly, Shamrock learned. He sparred with rookies and veterans alike, studying the intricate moves of submission fighting: armbars, kneebars, Achilles locks, chokes. The veteran fighters had all been exposed to the best of various martial arts, including muay Thai, karate, and judo. This was a new world for Shamrock, a world where strength mattered, but technique mattered more. Shamrock realized he was a gifted and talented fighter, but one who was incomplete. He absorbed the fundamentals of submission fighting with the zeal of a religious convert.

In America, Shamrock had learned to wrestle, to brawl, to rumble. In Japan, he learned to fight with finesse.

During his first year in Japan, Shamrock fought for the Universal Wrestling Federation, a professional wrestling circuit. The pro wrestlers in Japan are tough, well-conditioned fighters with a wealth of skill and technique. In the main, Japanese fans like their action realistic, not comedic. But even with the UWF, most matches were worked, or choreographed, the outcomes pre-determined.

Athletic, supremely self-confident, now versed in submissions technique, Shamrock began searching for something more challenging, more real. He found it with a group known as Pancrase, a reality-based breakaway from the UWF. Founded by Funaki and a group of Japanese businessmen, Pancrase was named after the pancration fights of the ancient Olympics. In Pancrase tournaments, no closed-fist strikes or headbutts were to be allowed. The fights would feature kicks, palm strikes, joint locks, and chokes. Most of the matches would go to the canvas and stress ground technique. A fight could be restarted, with both fighters told to stand up, if one fighter grabs the rope.

As a Pancrase fighter, Shamrock mastered submissions, learned more about kicking and striking, and flourished. He became a fusion of power, technique, and unwavering mental focus. Within weeks of the first Pancrase program, Shamrock had beaten both Suzuki and Funaki. He gained a rabid following and was featured in an action comic book. He earned a contract with Pancrase as both a featured performer and a trainer to recruit and prepare American fighters for Pancrase competition.

Shamrock began a life that was both hectic and improbable.

He flew once a month to Tokyo for three or four days to fight, then returned to the quiet village of Lockeford, just outside Lodi, to train, to watch over Lion's Den, and tend to his growing family.

In September of 1993, one of Shamrock's students noticed an ad in a martial arts magazine calling for fighters to compete in an unusual pay-per-view event to be called the Ultimate Fighting Championship. Shamrock's father, Bob, called a Los Angeles adman named Art Davie who was helping stage the program. Based on his discussions with Davie, the elder Shamrock was convinced the event was legitimate, would actually happen, and would showcase his son's skills for the first time before an American TV audience. There would be a $1,000 check for the eight competitors; those advancing to the semi-finals would get $5,000; those moving to the final would make $15,000 if they lost, $50,000 if they won.

The fight was set for November 12th in Denver, Colorado, a state with no athletic commission, no legal mechanism to reject or even challenge the first televised bare-knuckle fighting tournament in the history of the country.

Training in Lodi, Shamrock felt sure he would claim the purse, but there was more at stake—much more. There would be reflective glory for Pancrase, new respect for submission fighting and Lion's Den. And there would be the certainty that Ken Shamrock was the best fighter in the world.

Though he had gained minor celebrity status in Japan, Shamrock remained a relative unknown in his home village of Lockeford and the nearby town of Lodi. That began to change with the announcement

that he would compete in an unorthodox fighting event to be presented nationwide. Shamrock was profiled in feature stories in both *The
(Stockton) Record,* the largest paper in San Joaquin County, as well as
the *Lodi News-Sentinel,* which serves the Lodi area. Both stories
appeared on page one, recounting the tale of Shamrock's unlikely rise
from delinquent to martial arts champion. "I vent my frustrations in a
positive way now," Shamrock told the *News-Sentinel.* In *The Record*
article, Tina Shamrock told of witnessing her husband's intensity. "He
has an ability to focus, to concentrate, that is almost scary," she said.

Though Bob Shamrock was convinced the daring bare-knuckle
production would take place, his son was not. "There had been lots of
talk about other freestyle tournaments and none had happened," he
said. "I figured this one would fizzle out, too." Shamrock was so skep-
tical about the UFC actually being staged that he agreed to fight in a
Pancrase match just five days before the Denver event.

The tournament did not fizzle, though. It exploded.

• • •

On the night of November 12, McNichols Arena in Denver was
charged with queasy anticipation. Hanging above the arena was a
banner, the logo of the new event, a man with a shaved head and a
massive, ungloved fists. At the center of the arena, ominous and prim-
itive, was a fighting pit in the shape of an octagon, a creative contri-
bution from Milius. The sinister octagon only added to the outlaw,
underground feel of the event. Would a man be maimed in this cage?
Even killed? Just what would happen here tonight, as powerful men
went after one another with no prohibitions save biting and eye-gouging? Was this, as the first critics charged, simple bloodsport?

Meyrowitz and his director, Michael Pillot, were on edge. "We
hadn't done this event before. *Nobody* had done this event before,"
Pillot said. "It was an experiment, and we were all just holding our
breaths."

Just twelve seconds into the first fight, the surprises began. A
Dutch kickboxer named Gerard Gordeau kicked 450-pound sumo
wrestler Telia Tuli flush in the mouth, sending one of Tuli's teeth
whizzing into the crowd. Tuli, bloodied and stunned, collapsed in a
fleshy heap on the canvas of the octagon. For a moment, the commentators seemed as stunned as the bloodied sumo wrestler. "The
tooth came out," deadpanned Jim Brown, the football legend. "Did
you catch that tooth?," asked Bill "Superfoot" Wallace. "No, I think

it ended up under the table somewhere," responded Kathy Long, an actress and kickboxer. "I'm going to find it later," Wallace said. "And I am going to get a dollar for it, just like I did when I was a kid."

The experiment continued. An amiable bruiser named Kevin Rosier hugged and slugged and finally stomped a game-but-winded Zane Frazier, until one of Frazier's seconds hurled a towel into the ring.

So far, there had been little of the technique, the martial savvy, that proponents had promised.

Finally, it was time for Shamrock's first fight. He had flown to Denver three days before from Tokyo, where he had choked out a fighter named Fuke in forty-four seconds. Shamrock knew nothing about any of his UFC opponents. Though somewhat surprised the event was coming off, he nonetheless felt ready to fight, ready to win. "I had been fighting in Japan for three years. I knew how to grapple. I knew submissions. I figured nobody there could take me," he said.

Tina Shamrock sat at the edge of the octagon. She had watched her husband fight only a few times, including the Toughman victories in North Carolina. Each time, she had seen the rage reborn. Each time, she had seen her husband prevail. Now she sat, excited and a little nervous, but expecting to witness her husband's finest hour.

Shamrock's first round opponent was Patrick Smith, a taekwondo heavyweight champion who boasted an astonishing if unsubstantiated record of 250–0. Smith, a Denver boy, was the hometown favorite. He was tall and fast and muscular, with menacing, maniac eyes. As Shamrock and his father strode to the octagon, Smith's entourage jeered at them. "You're gonna die!," shouted one. "You will be crushed!," warned another. Shamrock looked at Smith, who was glaring from inside the circle of assistants. "I will see you in the octagon," Shamrock said.

Shamrock entered the octagon alone, wearing a warm-up jacket and red Speedos over a metal cup. The Speedos are brief and tight, but they are not worn for style. They are like another skin, offering nothing to tug or pull or latch onto. Shamrock peeled off the black Pancrase warm-up jacket, and waited. His expression gave away absolutely nothing. His was the gamest of game faces, the jaw taut, the eyes like stilettos. In the seconds before a fight, Shamrock tries to make eye contact with his opponents. This is, in part, to show his opponent that he has absolutely no fear. It is also to probe the eyes of his adversary for jangling nerves, for anxiety, or for cool. What Shamrock sees in the eyes of the enemy can help dictate the pace or angle of his own attack.

As he looked into the roiled eyes of Patrick Smith, Shamrock knew Smith would be reckless, knew he would blast at him with the short-lived shriek of a Roman candle.

And that is precisely what Patrick Smith did, charging across the octagon and quickly trying to throw a kick at Shamrock's guts. Shamrock blocked the kick and hauled Smith to the canvas. He wrapped his arms around Smith to control him, and felt a body convulsed with adrenaline. Such a body, so taut and implosive, rapidly devours energy. "He was as hard and tight as a board," Shamrock said. "I could tell he was blowing up fast." Shamrock worked patiently, allowing his opponent to waste his stores of energy and concentration. When Shamrock knew the Roman candle was losing its heat, he moved decisively. And then it was over in a few seconds. Shamrock seized Smith's ankle, locked it under his armpit, and twisted it with a ferocity that might have left Smith in surgery. Smith, who had earlier boasted of his imperviousness to pain, quickly smashed the canvas in surrender.

It was yet another of the evening's surprises: a fight between two of the biggest, most buffed-out gladiators ended not with a dramatic blow or even a choke, but with a deftly twisted ankle.

Shamrock stood and lifted his arms in triumph, but Smith, apparently never before victimized by a submission hold, screamed his defiance. "I ain't hurt," he said. "Let's finish it." "It is finished," Shamrock said, walking away. "Enjoy the rest of the show."
Patrick Smith now boasted a record of 250–1.

It was only fourteen minutes until Shamrock's semi-final fight. His opponent was Rorion Gracie's younger brother, Royce, a ju-jitsu master. In his first fight, Gracie had taken on a boxer, Art Jimmerson, had thrown him to the ground and easily mounted him. Jimmerson, with no ground experience and burdened with twelve-ounce gloves, realized the futility of his position and tapped. He had not landed a single blow.

Shamrock had never heard of the Gracies, had never fought anyone with a gi, or canvas martial arts robe. But as he stood in the octagon and his eyes invaded those of the Brazilian, he saw composure, not panic. He knew Royce Gracie was not a fighter who would back off or burn out.

Yet Shamrock felt that by beating Smith he had already vanquished the toughest fighter of the tournament besides himself. Now he would claim his rightful prize, his vindication.

The men engaged and collapsed to the floor. Then began a scramble of gnarled, writhing limbs. Sensing a chance, an opening,

Shamrock rocked back to grab Gracie's ankle as he had Smith's. But Gracie coiled up over him, twining the sleeve of his gi under Shamrock's neck. Shamrock, seemingly unaware of the peril, continued his quest for Gracie's ankle. Gracie grabbed the sleeve of his gi and cinched it around Shamrock's throat. Shamrock, even before he felt pain, even before he felt his air passage closing down, pounded his hand to the floor.

But there was another surprise. Amazingly, the referee did not see the tap-out. He was puzzled by the sudden cessation of movement. "Continue," he exhorted the men. Shamrock, the competitive fires still blazing, might have lunged at Gracie, might have hammered him with a right hand. Might have yet won the fight. But he knew that would not be fair, not be right. He had surrendered. Gracie had won. "It is over," Shamrock told the referee. "I tapped."

Shamrock stood and offered his hand to Gracie. "Good job," Gracie said. "You are very strong." Inside, Shamrock was reeling. This was to be his showcase event, his breakthrough victory. Inexplicably, he had given up before feeling pain or the constriction of his airway. He had been lulled and beaten by a man he thought would be a relatively simple conquest.

This is not real, Shamrock thought to himself, in the center of the octagon before a television audience of perhaps three million people. This cannot be real. And then Shamrock felt something he had not before, and has not since. He felt himself floating above the Octagon, looking down at a man who was not Kenneth Wayne Shamrock at all, but a farce. An impostor.

Shamrock stepped from the octagon, managed a quick interview, and fled to his dressing room.

At ringside, Tina Shamrock was trembling. She had never seen her husband beaten, dominated by another man. He had always been the predator, never the prey. He was so strong, so fierce, so protective. She had always felt so safe around him, so secure. Like her husband, she was experiencing feelings she had never felt before. Tina Shamrock felt so vulnerable now, so terribly vulnerable.

Gracie went on to beat Gordeau, a composed and classy fighter, in the final match of the first Ultimate Fighting Championship. As he did with Shamrock, the Brazilian worked for position, found an opening, and rapidly applied a rear choke on the Dutchman.

So the winner of the first televised no-holds-barred tournament in America was not some strapping stud with a right hand like a pile driver. He was not a Chuck Norris-type striker and kicker, a whirling dervish of menace. Nor was he a Bruce Lee stylist, with flashy moves and quirky grunts and shouts. To all but the martial arts cognoscenti, the victor was a surprise; a Brazilian, at 178 pounds, the smallest man in the tournament, a skilled and stealthy fighter who took his prey to the ground and choked them like an anaconda. In this and the hundreds of reality tournaments to follow, most of the featured fights would be won or lost on the mat.

At the end, Jim Brown, whose legend was football, not martial arts, offered the most incisive comment of the night: "What we have learned here is that fighting is not what we thought it was."

Meyrowitz and Pillot exhaled. Save a dislodged tooth, there had been no maiming, certainly no butchery. The show had its rough spots, but it went as smoothly as a radical experiment could be expected to. And Meyrowitz, in the days to come, would discover one last surprise: his show was a hit. He would later buy out Davie and Gracie and own this event, this confluence of gladiators. Besides the proceeds from the global money machine, he would enjoy revenue from sizable live gates, from merchandise, from videotape rentals. Months after Denver, he would tell an interviewer he had been prosperous even before the UFC. "I *was* rich," he said. "I'm getting richer."

At a cocktail party just hours after the first UFC in Denver, all of the fighters and their entourages gathered. Royce Gracie, smiling broadly, accepted a mock check the size of a screen door for $50,000 from Art Davie. He was also given a silver medallion as the first ultimate fighter.

Ken and Tina Shamrock attended the party. Shamrock had regained his sense of balance, but he remained humiliated. Gracie was generous to him, even pulling him close and telling him, "you slipped. You could have won. It was a good fight."

For Shamrock, it was not even close to being a good fight.

As he watched Gracie accept the accolades, he made a vow to himself: I will beat that man. I will someday stand where that man is now. I will be back.

Chapter 9

Phantom

Grady Cole Arena
Charlotte, North Carolina
September 9, 1994

K en Shamrock stopped abruptly at the edge of the lights and the artificial mist. Somehow, this was not right. He was in the finals of the UFC. He was only yards from the octagon, only seconds from near-certain victory and a prize of $60,000.

Still, it was not right.

Royce Gracie had pulled out. And Royce Gracie was the man Shamrock wanted. The *only* man Shamrock wanted.

It had been nearly a year since Gracie had slipped behind Shamrock and choked him, shamed him in the first UFC. When he returned to Lodi from Denver after the tournament, Shamrock languished for days in a funk. He did not want to watch a tape of the fight, did not want to discuss it. He did not, truth be told, really want to leave the cocoon of his own home. Yet he did, over weeks, emerge from the malaise and the self-imposed isolation. And as he ascended from the depths, Shamrock renewed the promise he had made to himself in Denver to return to the octagon. To one day dominate the man who had stripped him, in a very real sense, of his dignity.

Shamrock planned to extract his revenge in the second UFC, set in March 1994 again in Denver. As with the first UFC, the winner would claim a substantial cash prize. But Shamrock would have fought for nothing. "He was determined to fight Royce again, whether it was in the octagon, in a dojo, or in a parking lot," Bob Shamrock said. "He wanted the rematch at all costs."

The only way to insure victory in the rematch, Shamrock knew, was to learn, to adapt, to become an even more complete and dangerous fighter. He had gone to Japan thinking he was invincible and he had been humiliated. Yet he had learned, progressed. Eventually, he had triumphed.

He went to Denver thinking he was invincible and once again he was defeated. Again, he would learn. And again, he felt, he would

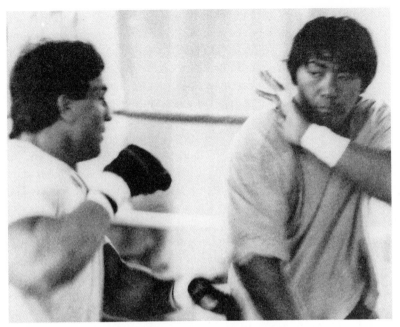

After losing in his first UFC, Shamrock redoubled his commitment to training and sparring. Here he is working at the Lion's Den with Masakatsu Funaki, one of the founders and leading fighters of Pancrase. *(Calixtro Romias photo)*

triumph. Shamrock is not a man of arts and letters. But he is a man who is convinced of the emancipating power of knowledge. At his Lion's Den dojo, he has always preached the fundamental value of submissions technique. But he has also stressed the need to take the best from other fighting styles. To refine and expand, to constantly absorb new information. "The day you stop learning," he said, "is the day you should quit." Shamrock lectures his students intensively on the fundamentals of submissions, on the chokes and joint locks that most often end a fight between skilled fighters. But he makes certain his students are efficient strikers and kickers as well. He shows them how to make clean, explosive takedowns. The goal, Shamrock said, is to be conditioned, mentally tough and technically flawless. Though he is the unquestioned master of submissions at the Lion's Den, he brings in guest lecturers, including Maurice Smith, U.S. heavyweight kickboxing champion and an Extreme Fighting champion, to help his fighters—and himself—become even more skilled.

Oddly, in his Toughmans, in his bar brawls and fist fights for money and in his matches in Japan, Shamrock had never fought a man with a gi. He was aware a gi could be a weapon for the man wearing it as well as a burden. He knew he must now learn more about the gi and more about ju-jitsu. And more about this Gracie family that seemed to practice the art with such finesse.

Shamrock viewed videotapes of ju-jitsu stylists and traveled to a ju-jitsu studio in Los Angeles. He learned the Gracies, though relative newcomers to the United States, were folk heroes in their native country of Brazil.

The story of the Gracies, in fact, is among the most colorful in modern martial arts. The family gained the secrets of ju-jitsu from Japanese champion Esai Maeda just after the turn of the century. The Asian master had traveled to Brazil to help establish a Japanese immigrant colony. He was assisted in the venture by a man named Gastao Gracie, a Brazilian scholar and politician of Scottish descent. To repay Gracie for his help, Maeda taught Gracie's son, Carlos, ju-jitsu techniques that had never been used before on the Latin American continent. Carlos, in turn, shared the techniques with his four brothers, including Helio Gracie, who is the father of Royce and Rorion. (In Portuguese, Rs are pronounced much like Hs. So Royce is "Hoyce," Rorion is "Horion," and Rickson, another brother, is properly pronounced "Hickson." Helio believes the letter R has magical qualities, thus all nine of his children have names starting with the letter.)

Helio weighed only 140 pounds in his fighting prime, but he was both supremely analytical and tenacious. He began reinventing the techniques shared by Maeda so they could be used effectively by men of all sizes and weight classes.

Starting in his teens, Helio began winning battles against much larger and more experienced opponents, eventually challenging anyone in Brazil to a no-holds-barred fight to the finish. There were few takers. Helio did fight the Japanese champion Kato and choked him out. In 1951, Helio fought another Japanese ju-jitsu master, Masahiko Kimura. Thousands of Brazilian fans jammed the Maracana Stadium to witness the fight, which Kimura won with a choke after thirteen minutes. It was hardly a bitter defeat. Helio Gracie was forty-two years old at the time, Kimura thirty-four. Helio was outweighed by Kimura, perhaps the finest Japanese martial artist of the century, by more than fifty pounds.

Gracie challenged many of the great boxers of his era, including Joe Louis. All politely declined to wage war against the diminutive but crafty Brazilian.

The Gracie male offspring have all been immersed in ju-jitsu, Helio-style. The family's subtle fighting techniques were brought to the United States in 1979 by Rorion Gracie. Rorion cleaned houses in Bel Aire and Brentwood during the day and taught chokes and armbars in his garage in Torrance at night. He met a movie producer who offered him a job as fight consultant for the movie *Lethal Weapon* and orchestrated the hand-to-hand showdown between Mel Gibson and Gary Busey in the film. It was, in retrospect, a huge break. Later, Rorion met Chuck Norris and shared with him ju-jitsu moves Norris used in the movie, *Hero and the Terror.*

Demand for Rorion's ju-jitsu instruction became so great that in 1984 he called little brother Royce up from Brazil to help out. In the first year, Royce spent most of his time babysitting the children of Rorion and Suzanne Gracie and trying to pick up English. Eventually he was a lead instructor at the new Gracie Ju-jitsu Academy in Torrance. When Rorion became one of the founders of the UFC, Royce Gracie volunteered to carry the family's tradition into the event.

And so the prowess displayed by Royce Gracie in the octagon was the product of an unlikely cultural passage spanning more than a millennium. Jujitsu was developed in India, exported to China, refined in Japan, then taken to Brazil, where it was fine-tuned by Brazilians of Scottish heritage and finally, in the form reinvented by the Gracies, brought to the United States.

Shamrock was impressed by the Gracie fighting tradition, but not awed by it. He saw Gracie-style ju-jitsu as an opportunistic art relying to a large degree on a blunder by the opponent. Shamrock had blundered when he had turned his back on Gracie while stalking Gracie's ankle. He had blundered when he failed to detect the danger of Gracie's gi slipping under his chin.

He noticed aspects of the Gracie's approach he felt he could exploit. Because they were compact, the Gracies were not eager to duke it out with a heavy-fisted opponent. In fact, they did everything they could to keep from getting hit. The gi could be useful, no doubt. The sleeve could be wedged toward an opponent's windpipe and yanked tight like a noose. The cuff could be grasped to hold an opponent's arm or leg, like a third hand. The thick canvas of the gi, rubbed across an opponent's face or neck, could chafe the skin like a rasp. It could also absorb moisture form an opponent's sweat-slickened limbs, making it easier to apply a hold.

But the gi could also be a liability, especially in a long fight when it would only intensify the heat and discomfort of its owner. While the

Gracies were in good condition, they were not, Shamrock felt, exceptionally strong or durable. Shamrock returned to Lodi with a battle plan. He would use power against Gracie. He would land dozens if not hundreds of punishing blows. He would prepare for a long, ugly siege of a fight. And he would not blunder into an easy choke.

Shamrock trained relentlessly for the showdown, forcing his sparring partners to wear gis and come at him with the ju-jitsu moves he had discovered on his recent fact-finding mission. Shamrock ran, jumped rope, lifted weights, and sparred with unprecedented determination. He would be prepared, he said, to fight for an hour or two or even three. "Whatever it takes," he said.

And Shamrock would not try to squeeze in a Pancrase match the same week as his upcoming UFC fight, as he had before. He was singularly focused on defeating Royce Gracie, on reclaiming his pride.

Then, just three weeks before the UFC, sparring with one of his students, Shamrock reached up to block a kick. He felt something snap in his right hand. Later, the doctor held up the X-ray and told Shamrock what he already suspected: the hand was fractured and would have to be set in a cast. Initially, Shamrock refused, saying he could not afford a cast to be placed on his hand, could not afford to miss what might be the fight of his life. "Then you will likely suffer a compound fracture," the doctor replied. "And this next fight will probably be the last of your career." Shamrock, thinking of his family, thinking of the long term, reluctantly allowed the plaster to be wrapped around the hand. In the next few weeks, though, the rage would rise, and Royce Gracie would appear in his mind's eye as a phantom, a phantom who was retreating into the distance. More than once, Shamrock fought the urge to simply shatter the cast, remove it, and stride into the octagon.

Shamrock did fly to Denver for the UFC, where he was interviewed at ringside by a commentator. But then Shamrock sat and smoldered and watched Gracie win the Ultimate Fighting Championship II.

Given time, Shamrock's hand healed and the UFC organizers, still convinced of Shamrock's popularity, included him in the third version of what was becoming a very lucrative franchise.

The event, set in Charlotte, was billed as a grudge match. Shamrock and Gracie posed for publicity photos together. One was blown up into a billboard and dangled over Sunset Boulevard, the two men clinched, staring coldly into each other's eyes.

Despite growing criticism by some who felt it was too violent, the event was staged as planned in Charlotte's Grady Cole Arena.

Meyrowitz and company had fine-tuned the production. Instead of a bleak, sanitized white, the floor of the octagon was now a pleasing sky blue. Instead of the Brazilian officials who clumsily presided over the first event, organizers had recruited as referee John McCarthy, a Los Angeles cop and martial artist who stands 6'6". No longer was a bell sounded to commence each fight; just McCarthy's command to "get it on." There was one more change, this one a testament to the infamous flying tooth of Telia Tuli. Mouthpieces were now mandatory for all fighters.

With Shamrock and Gracie both in the tournament, and obviously the class of the field, it seemed a near-certainty the two would meet in the final. And the tournament progressed according to form before 5,000 rabid fans in Grady Cole—for the first twenty minutes.

Shamrock faced Christophe Leininger from Scottsdale, Arizona, a member of the U.S. National Judo Team, a game and talented fighter. Shamrock was confident, but also very concerned. Like Gracie, Leininger wore a gi. Unlike Gracie, Leininger was powerfully built and might throw some telling blows. "The fight was a test, my first time back in the UFC," Shamrock said. "I wondered how I would do against another fighter in a gi, especially a guy as tough and experienced as Leininger." Shamrock's strength was more than a match for Leininger's craft, as he tossed the judo man to the ground and climbed on top of him. With a massive upper-body and the balance of a gyroscope, Shamrock is very difficult to dislodge from either the mount or guard position. He hammered Leininger into a tap-out. The fight lasted four minutes, forty-eight seconds. Leininger, new to the UFC and to the fury and power of Ken Shamrock, conceded to him after the fight: "That was not what I expected."

The semi-final fight was not what Shamrock expected. He faced an alternate, a man named Felix Lee Mitchell, a Tennessee prison guard and kung-fu champion. As an alternate, Mitchell had not fought yet, not even broken a sweat. His freshness and power surprised Shamrock. He had to struggle mightily to drop Mitchell to the canvas and injured his knee in the effort. Mitchell's tactics surprised him, too. Near the end of the fight, Mitchell grabbed into Shamrock's Speedos and tried to dislodge his protective metal cup, then bang his fist into Shamrock's groin. The gambit failed, however, as the Speedos held Shamrock's protection tight. Shamrock was able to wear Mitchell down and choke him from behind. Yet Shamrock, weary, with an aching knee and miffed at Mitchell's unseemly groping, did not offer his customary handshake after the fight. Limping slightly, he returned to his dressing room and waited for his showdown with a phantom. He had made the finals.

Royce Gracie, though, was having problems of his own, problems that dwarfed those faced by Shamrock.

In his first round, Gracie had drawn a wild card, a large and well-muscled Hawaiian brawler with a trace of taekwondo experience named Kimo Leopoldo. Leopoldo, who goes by simply "Kimo," is a reformed drug addict and street hustler. He is also a born again Christian who claims he fights to help spread the gospel of Jesus Christ. Before the fight, Kimo's manager, a shrill and annoying man named Joe San, told an interviewer from *Details* magazine, "don't get in the ring with Kimo if you do not have Jesus in your heart. You might die." The pony-tailed Kimo walked into the arena wearing a shroud and lugging a big wooden cross on his shoulders.

He was clearly not the typical UFC gladiator. His fight with odds-on favorite Royce Gracie was not typical, either.

Kimo, in fact, could and probably should have won the fight. He surged across the octagon and took the battle to Gracie, throwing a barrage of erratic punches and remaining on his feet despite Gracie's best efforts to drag him away from the fenced side of the octagon to the canvas. Finally, the two spun to the floor, with Kimo behind Gracie, riding his back—in the perfect position for a rear choke. Relatively unschooled in submissions, Kimo could not set the choke. So the melee continued, with Gracie grabbing Kimo's ponytail and controlling the bigger man's head with the knot of hair. Another roll, another missed chance for a choke by Kimo, and Gracie was finally able to capture the Hawaiian's left arm between his legs and apply an armbar. Utterly spent, Kimo could barely muster the tap out necessary to end what had been the most exciting fight of the evening. It had been a little more than five minutes of mayhem. Gracie gimped out of the arena, his arms draped on the shoulders of his brothers, his gi spattered with blood, his eyes downcast.

The semi-final fight would match Gracie and Harold Howard, a husky, bearded blonde Canadian, to determine who would advance to face Shamrock in the final. The intense Howard, a black belt in karate, marched briskly into the octagon and bounced in place, looking loose and confident. In contrast, Gracie shuffled slowly into the octagon. Haggard, still slathered in sweat, his head still hung low, a bandage under his left eye, the pride of the Gracie clan looked like the victim of a car wreck. He did not face Howard, but instead drooped against the chain link of the octagon. Clearly, Gracie could not fight now.

And Helio Gracie, the 82-year-old patriarch, standing just inches from his suffering son, performed an act of both compassion and courage, considering his family's magnificent fighting tradition. He took the white towel from around his shoulders and threw it to the center of the octagon. Gracie had surrendered. Howard would advance to the finals of UFC III to face Ken Shamrock.

So now Shamrock stood in the artificial mist, on the precipice, his knee aching, wondering what he was doing in this place, at this time. What would he prove, fighting Harold Howard, a large and game fighter, but a relative amateur? Shamrock was a professional. He had prepared, he had hungered, to fight another professional, a man name Gracie. Now there was nothing to prove. No reason to test his injured knee further. His pride had been stripped by Gracie, not the golden-haired Canadian.

He looked at his father. "I can't do it," he said.

Organizers moved swiftly. They notified alternate fighter Steve Jennum that he would face Howard in the final. And the crew-cut Jennum took the much larger Howard to the floor of the octagon, straddled him, and pounded him bloody. The winner of UFC III and $60,000 was an unknown cop from Omaha.

Again, the phantom had eluded Ken Shamrock.

Chapter 10

Redemption

Lodi
April, 1995

S hamrock's father refused to speak to him for two days. When he
did speak, the words were not soothing. Father rebuked son for
not finishing the battle, for not meeting his responsibilities, for
backing up when he should have stepped forward. "You have been
fighting to control the rage all your life," he said. "You could have
used the rage for five more minutes and then snuffed it out."

Shamrock weathered his father's blistering words and remained
unconvinced. The decision not to fight in the finals of UFC III, he still
believed, was the right one. In his mind, the fight against Howard
would have been neither fair nor right. He had mowed through two
other fighters to get to Gracie. He saw no reason to mow down a third
for the mere sport of it.

Besides, it appeared that the phantom would finally be his. His
alone. Meyrowitz and Davie, aware fans still thirsted to see a
Shamrock-Gracie rematch, developed a new format to make sure it
would happen. They called it a Superfight. It would be a one-on-one
marquee contest to precede the championship fight of the tournament. There would be no danger of these premier fighters being elim-
inated through injury or exhaustion. They would face only each other,
no one else. The first Superfight would match Ken Shamrock against
Royce Gracie.

Shamrock was elated. He redoubled his commitment to training,
refocusing on a long, patient fight during which he would steadily
pound away at Gracie and avoid making any mistakes.

The fight was held in Charlotte, North Carolina on April 15,
1995. Shamrock was in the best condition of his life, physically and
mentally. The knee had healed quickly, so quickly that Shamrock
fought in and won a major Pancrase tournament in Tokyo in
December. After facing and beating four opponents in two days,
including Maurice Smith and Masa Funaki, he was officially crowned
the King of Pancrase. Now, Shamrock believed, he would add the

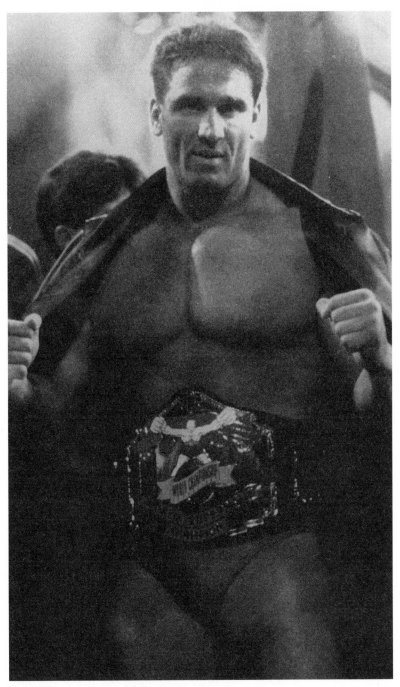

Shamrock claimed the Superfight belt with a victory over Dan Severn in Caspar, Wyoming. *(SEG photo)*

UFC Superfight title and be the undisputed bare-knuckle champion of both Asia and the United States.

At the managers' meeting the night before the fight in Charlotte, the Gracie and Shamrock camps were respectful. "Hello my friend," said Bob Shamrock, embracing Helio Gracie. "Hello, Bob," Helio said. "It will be a great fight. I am just glad I am not the one fighting Ken."

Helio Gracie was right. It was a great fight, though most of the 8,000 fans in Charlotte did not understand that.

At McCarthy's signal, Shamrock and Gracie moved to the center of the octagon. Gracie popped some quick kicks toward Shamrock's thighs, a common ju-jitsu technique to keep an opponent at bay and gauge the distance for a shoot and takedown. Shamrock tossed a hard right that just missed, then he shot into the eggshell gi of Royce Gracie and took him cleanly to the ground. Gracie was on the bottom, Shamrock on the top in the guard position. And there, for many long minutes, they remained. Gracie tried to peck his heels into Shamrock's kidneys. Shamrock did not flinch. Gracie tried to chip at Shamrock's neck with rabbit punches. Shamrock was oblivious. As the fight ground on, Shamrock, in black Speedos and black Asics wrestling shoes, began the assault. He banged at Gracie's ribs with short, telling punches. When Gracie pulled his hands down to protect his ribs, Shamrock threw slashing palm strikes to his face. He rammed his knee into Gracie's tailbone. He launched headbutts into Gracie's chin, his cheek, his forehead. Most important, he did not rush, did not make a mistake.

The Charlotte crowd wanted heavy strikes, quick movement, dramatic kicks. Instead, they were getting a sweat-soaked chess match. A few fans began hurling boos toward the octagon. Even Bob Shamrock was growing restive. "Get up and punch him!," he told his son. "Get up and do something."

Shamrock, though, knew precisely what he was doing. He continued his steady siege. At thirty-one minutes, six seconds, McCarthy stood the fighters up. There would be a five minute overtime. The fighters again moved toward one another, Gracie again flicking out the thigh-checks. And then the man who had won three Toughman competitions with the power of his fists threw a straight right hand at Gracie and nailed him flush in the right eye. Stunned, Gracie tumbled down, Shamrock on top of him. It was Shamrock's opening, his opportunity. He clicked up the pace, launched headbutts at Gracie's rapidly swelling eye, threw punch after punch at his face. The crowd, suddenly enlivened, began to chant, *"Shamrock! Shamrock! Shamrock!"*

Gracie, somehow, managed to hang on and survive the siege. The first Superfight ended after 36 minutes, six seconds. It was the longest fight in the short history of the UFC.

With no judges at ringside, the contest was listed as a draw. But it was a moral and strategic victory for Shamrock, who had used power and patience to dominate Gracie, dominate the phantom who would haunt him no more. Gracie stood slowly, his face a puffed and purple mask. "Royce Gracie is a mess—but Ken Shamrock looks marvelous," said Bruce Beck, one of the television commentators. Shamrock stood and raised his hands high, looking like he could fight for another hour, or two. Whatever it might take.

Gracie was reportedly rushed to a hospital for an examination of his bloated eye. He later appeared at the after-fight party, saying little, wearing dark sunglasses that shielded his wounds. He left after perhaps five minutes. Shamrock, meanwhile, luxuriated in the affection granted a newly crowned king. He signed autographs and posed for photos and accepted the congratulations of Meyrowitz and Davie. The fight had not provided the clear-cut triumph he had hoped and worked for. But it was redemption nonetheless.

Organizers badly wanted another rematch between Shamrock and Gracie. The Gracies balked. Shamrock was too big, they said. He would have to lose thirty pounds for Royce to fight him again. Shamrock agreed to drop fifteen pounds, to establish his weight at about 200, but any lower would be absurd for a man of Shamrock's build. "They would like me to go to 175," Shamrock told friends. "I haven't weighed that since I was a junior in high school. And I have no intention of reliving my youth." The Gracies also resisted a time limit of thirty or even forty-five minutes. It takes time to wear down a large opponent like Shamrock, they maintained, ignoring the fact that as the Superfight ground on it was Gracie, not Shamrock, who was dissolving. And as the Gracies well knew, a fight with no time limit would be an impossibility on pay-per-view television. Finally, the Gracies wanted much, much more money to fight than had every been paid to a UFC competitor.

As the talks unraveled, it was clear the Gracies wanted nothing more to do with Ken Shamrock.

With Gracie declining to enter the octagon again, UFC promoters decided the man to face Shamrock in the next Superfight would be the winner of the last UFC tournament. His name: Dan Severn.

Severn is a massive wrestler with God-given strength. "He is genetically big. His arms are big, his legs are big, his hands are big," said Phyliss Lee, Severn's former manager. "He was always complaining about how they couldn't make weight machines strong enough for him, that he would break them." Severn was an outstanding high school wrestler in Michigan and earned a full-ride athletic scholarship to Arizona State University. After graduation, he continued to compete off-and-on while working as a coach both in Arizona and in Michigan. Severn dreamed of winning an Olympic medal, but that never happened. He began selling wrestling gear, singlets and shoes and shorts. Through the years he continued to stay in reasonably good shape and even competed now and again, winning senior amateur tournaments. He toiled in relative obscurity, selling merchandise, wrestling a little, coaching a little, hoping to extract something from his talent before his body gave out. At age thirty-six, he met Lee, a savvy and veteran pro-wrestling manager based in Ohio. "I kind of felt sorry for Dan, to tell you the truth," she said. "He was an older guy who had been around for a while and had invested so much of his life in wrestling. But he had nothing to show for it." Lee agreed to line up some pro-wrestling spots for Severn. Watching the big man in the ring, though, Lee felt he would not find much success there, either. "He had no fan appeal," she said. "He was just big and dull." Lee decided there was just one place left for Severn to try and seek his glory: the controversial world of reality combat.

"We knew he was an experienced wrestler, that he was big and strong," Lee said. "The only question was whether he was willing to go into the octagon and do what he had to do to win."

He was. Severn proved himself a methodical if not stylish competitor, sweeping through UFC V, defeating Joe Charles, Oleg Taktarov, and David Beneteau. Severn was not an exceptional puncher or kicker. But using his size and know-how, he could take men to the ground and dominate them, grind them, maul them into submission or to the point McCarthy felt obliged to end the fight. He even won a nickname from SEG executives: "The Beast."

He was finally gaining the fortune and acclaim he had struggled for much of his life. He had done so well in the UFC that he became convinced no one, including Ken Shamrock, could beat him, said Lee. Before the Superfight, set July 14 in Casper, Wyoming, Severn sent confidential letters to several friends predicting exactly how he would defeat Shamrock. "Dan, in my mind, was overconfident," Lee said. "Writing that letter was the wrong thing to do." He was also becoming something of a prima donna. When he arrived in Casper three days before the event, Severn learned Shamrock was already ensconced at the hotel and had been for nearly a week. He threw a tantrum, Lee said, accusing SEG of favoring Shamrock, of granting him an early advantage for training and lodgings in Casper. What Severn did not know is that Shamrock, having learned the hard lesson of his first UFC in Denver, was now arranging to arrive at the fight location up to ten days before the actual event. This gave him time to focus, to find a proper training center, to become accustomed to the elevation and climate of the city. He did this at his own expense.

Severn also insinuated that Shamrock's success was in part due to using steroids. Though Shamrock had experimented with steroids years before as a pro wrestler, he had not used them in either Pancrase or UFC competition. Shamrock, like Severn, possessed natural, God-given strength, which he increased with tough hours or sparring and weightlifting. Severn's aspersions, offered without a whit of evidence, angered Shamrock, increasingly sensitive to his position as a father and role model.

Shamrock was starting to view Severn as not just an opponent, but an antagonist.

During a pre-fight press conference in Casper, Shamrock patiently listened as Severn and other fighters offered their comments. When Shamrock began speaking, Severn abruptly rose and left the room. Shamrock felt the rage rise in his veins. His eyes shot fire at Lee, who remained in the room. "Before, I was just going to beat him," Shamrock growled. "Now I am going to hurt him." Lee, seldom at a loss for words, retorted: "In your dreams."

The Casper fans, many sporting cowboy hats, hooted and yelped as Shamrock and Severn faced off in the center of the octagon for the contest, billed as "The Clash of the Titans."

Many UFC fans, like Severn himself, were convinced he would prevail over Shamrock; an informal Internet survey conducted the evening of the event showed fifty-five percent of those responding favored Severn, thirty-nine percent favored Shamrock, and six-percent were unsure. Apparently some felt Severn, the heavier man by forty pounds, would take Shamrock down and smother him as he had his other opponents. But Severn had never faced a man with the intricate arsenal of Ken Shamrock. And Shamrock, a fanatic for preparation, had spotted a weakness in Severn's technique: the wrestler, time and again, dropped his head low as he dove in to lasso his opponent's legs for a take-down. Severn, though a powerful and accomplished grappler, would be vulnerable to what is known as a guillotine choke, Shamrock felt.

The two clinched, engaged, remained on their feet. It appeared to be a classic Greco-Roman wrestling match. Severn tried to hook and jerk Shamrock to the ground, but he could not. Severn then tried to shoot in on Shamrock. As Shamrock expected, Severn's head drooped low. Shamrock wrapped his arm around Severn's thickly muscled neck. Using the bone in his forearm, Shamrock searched for Severn's Adam's apple, knowing a choke planted there would bring excruciating pain and a quick tap-out. But Severn managed to torque his gigantic body away from the forearm, away from danger. The two tied up again. Then Severn dove down once more to trap Shamrock's legs, and inexplicably, once more dropped his head low. This time, there would be no escape. Shamrock instantly snared his arm around Severn's head. He would not bother to probe for the Adam's apple this time but would patiently tighten the circle of flesh and bone around the neck of Dan Severn. The noose tightened, steadily tightened. Like a soda straw bent in half, Severn's windpipe was closing down, the air flow to his brain shutting off. Severn, desperate now and slumping to the floor, threw a wild punch at Shamrock's groin and missed. And then, helpless and beaten and rapidly hurtling toward unconsciousness, Severn dropped his hand on the canvas. It had taken only two-minutes, thirteen-seconds. A jubilant Ken Shamrock was presented with the glittering Superfight belt.

Afterward, Severn again shared his suspicion with Phyliss Lee about Shamrock and steroids. "He said Shamrock was much, much stronger than he expected," Lee said. "Dan said he had never fought a man before who he couldn't move. He said he couldn't move Shamrock."

Severn did not know it at the time, but he would be given another chance at the man possessing the astonishing strength, the man who had battled his way to become the first King of Pancrase. And now become the first-ever Superfight champion of the UFC.

Chapter 11

Bare Knuckles

Los Angeles
December 6, 1995

S ome call it ultimate fighting," said Larry King, well-known CNN talk show host. "And some call it the ultimate in brutality." King had decided to explore the building controversy over reality fighting events, the most prominent being the Ultimate Fighting Championship. "We'll look at a frightening new fad that might be coming to *your* town," King told his viewers.

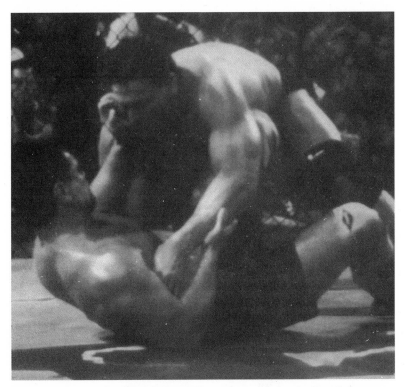

With controversy about the UFC building, Shamrock fought Oleg Taktarov (on his back) in a Superfight in Buffalo, N.Y. After the event, efforts to regulate the event, led by Sen. John McCain of Arizona, intensified. *(SEG photo)*

King's guests included Senator John McCain from Arizona, Bob Meyrowitz, Marc Ratner, executive director of the Nevada Athletic Commission, and Superfight champion Ken Shamrock. King, McCain and Meyrowitz were in King's Washington D.C. studio, Ratner was beamed in from Las Vegas, and Shamrock from Los Angeles.

McCain, a former prisoner of war in Vietnam and a staunch Republican, had emerged as the point man in the campaign to stop the UFC and other freestyle fighting events.

An old friend of King's, the senator smiled confidently when introduced on the set. The senator looked like a man who expected to claim easy victory in this, the most visible exchange to date on the merits of reality combat. With his silver hair, the senator was handsome, telegenic. And clearly, McCain felt he held the high moral ground in this discussion. The smile, though, would not last.

Since the first UFC in Denver, critics howling "savagery," had called for its prohibition. McCain, a boxer in high school and at the Naval Academy, and still an avid boxing fan, had urged governors to block the event, warning that the UFC posed, "an unacceptable risk to the lives and health of the contestants." Syndicated columnist George Will joined the high-minded crusade, writing that, "participants in these events are frightening, but less so than the paying customers. They include slack-jawed children whose parents must be cretins, and raving adults."

The debate over Ultimate Fighting had historical roots. In the 1800s, the political aristocracy rose up against the increasingly popular sport of bare-knuckle prizefighting. John L. Sullivan, "The Boston Boy," is remembered as the country's first great boxer. He was also a convict and a fugitive, a man who fought on barges and in secret locations in marshes and sand dunes to elude arrest. After winning a critical victory 1898 in Richburg, Mississipi, for instance, Sullivan was spirited

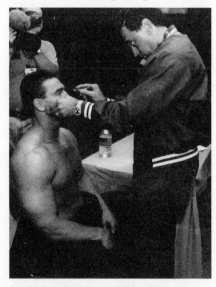

Dr. Richard Istrico of New York, the UFC's chief physician, examines Shamrock before a UFC event. *(Calixtro Romias photo)*

out of the deep South and safely returned to New York City. But the governor of Mississippi succeeded in having an arrest warrant served on Sullivan and the champion was transported back to Mississippi for trial. The journey to Mississippi revealed the growing gap between populace and politician: at each train stop, thousands gathered to cheer Sullivan. In Jackson, the capital city, the bare-knuckle king was celebrated at a gala reception. At a court hearing in Purvis, Mississippi, charges of prize fighting and assault and battery were eventually dropped, though Sullivan claimed later he had spent more in travel and legal expenses than he had cleared in the fight.

In a misguided attempt to dress up what they felt was an unseemly spectacle, critics in the 1890s did succeed in imposing the Marquis of Queensberry rules on organized prizefighting. Fighters would no longer be able to strike with their bare knuckles. Instead, their hands would be cloaked in padded gloves. The move prevented countless broken knuckles and staunched the flow of blood in the decades to come. But it also contributed to hundreds of deaths. The padded and gloved fist, thought to be more civilized, allowed fighters to repeatedly bash the heads of opponents and inflict unseen damage to the brain. Dr. Richard Istrico, the New York-based physician who is the UFC's chief medical advisor, puts it this way: "In bare knuckle fighting, you have some soft tissue trauma. A broken nose, bruising, some bleeding. But when you put a heavy glove on the fist, you have an increased risk of neurological trauma."

There are no definitive studies on the number of boxers killed worldwide since the adoption of the Marquis of Queensberry rules. But one study cited in a 1995 *Miami Harold* report suggested that at least 400 boxers had died of fight-related injuries since 1945; a 1995 *USA Today* piece said an average of four boxers a year die from head trauma suffered in the ring.

At the time of the Larry King broadcast, the UFC had staged nearly 100 fights. Blood had flowed, a tooth had been knocked lose, men had been rendered unconscious. There were heavy bruises, such as the one suffered by Gracie under his eye during his Superfight with Shamrock. Nearly all examples of what Istrico describes as soft-tissue trauma. There had been no lasting injuries, certainly no deaths. Nor had there been deaths in Japan or Brazil or Russia or other countries where such events had been staged.

Meyrowitz required fighters to sign a waiver holding him harmless in case of injury or death and critics pointed to the waiver as evidence of the event's fatal danger. Meyrowitz found the hue and cry amusing. "The waiver was based on the one I had to sign before I could play polo at my club," he said. The founder of the UFC, in fact, contended polo and even NCAA basketball posed more risk to the well-being of participants than his bare-knuckle clashes.

Meyrowitz and UFC producers held at least a measure of responsibility for the UFC's blood-smearing, bone-shattering reputation. After all, the first press release on the event called it a "rock 'em, sock 'em, hurt 'em," affair that would play out until "only one man remains standing."

While Meyrowitz, at least early-on, played up the raw action of his venture, he also took numerous precautions. "A guy walking into the octagon could stumble and break his neck. You just never know," he said. So the UFC regulated itself. Contestants had to submit blood tests, including HIV checks, along with MRI scans to reveal possible brain abnormalities. Fighters also underwent physical exams before they were accepted to fight in the octagon. Istrico provided another exam the day of the fight. McCarthy, the referee, had the full authority, which he regularly exercised, to stop a fight if a combatant could not defend himself. Competitors were examined in a so-called triage room after each match. Physicians with both neurological and orthopedic expertise were always on standby at the events, along with paramedics and ambulances.

The UFC would never be as safe as a croquet tournament. But neither would it pose the deceptive and deadly risks of a boxing event.

Not surprisingly, many boxers and boxing commissioners railed against the UFC and similar productions. It was in their financial and political interests to do so, of course: What would become of boxing if fans came to understand that mixed martial arts tournaments were not only frequently more entertaining, but safer?

Shamrock, the veteran of numerous wrestling matches and fist fights, of three Toughman tournaments, of Pancrase fights and UFC bouts, was convinced the UFC was as safe as it could be. Now, as he sat in a Los Angeles television studio, he was the undisputed human embodiment of the UFC.

After defeating Severn, Shamrock had retained his Superfight belt with a draw in September 1995 against Oleg Taktarov in Buffalo, New York. Taktarov is a tough, battle-tested Russian who boasts a remarkable background. Taktarov grew up in Siberia and served with the Russian military. Assigned to a remote forest outpost, Taktarov said, he one day felt a horrible pain rise in his gut. His commander refused his request to leave for medical help. Sensing a life-threatening condition,

Taktarov left anyway and struggled to a country hospital several miles away. The attending physician diagnosed critical appendicitis and told Taktarov he had no more than twenty minutes to live. He operated, and, Taktarov recalled, saved his life. Later, in retribution for bolting from his outpost, Taktarov claims he was sent to Afghanistan. He refused to kill civilians, though, and was sent to a military lock-up for a time. He later trained an elite division of the KGB in hand-to-hand combat and, after leaving the military, won national sambo and ju-jitsu tournaments.

After arriving in the United States, he befriended Guy Mezger, one of the Lion's Den fighters. Mezger, in turn, introduced Taktarov to Shamrock, who allowed him to stay at his fighter's home in Lockeford and train at the Lion's Den for Pancrase fights in Japan.

During their fight in Buffalo, Shamrock tried to strike Taktarov enough to force McCarthy to stop the fight. He landed numerous blows, but Taktarov did not tap out and was never in grave enough danger for McCarthy to intervene. Though the fight would be recorded as a draw, most observers felt Shamrock dominated the Russian and would have handily won a judge's decision if judges had been in place.

Shamrock, wearing a grey sports jacket and black sport shirt, looked cool and relaxed as Larry King began the discussion on the UFC. As he listened to McCain, though, he became alarmed by the senator's obvious lack of understanding about the UFC and reality fighting. As the program continued, Shamrock, not McCain, would be the most outspoken and arguably the most incisive participant.

"So what's the rub, senator?," asked King.

"Well, some of this is so brutal that it is just nauseating," McCain said. "It appeals to the lowest common denominator in our society. This is something I think there is no place for . . . this emphasizes blood and crippling a combatant."

Ratner, executive director of the Nevada State Athletic Commission, agreed with McCain and pointed out the UFC would never gain the approval of his commission because, "it is just too violent. In boxing, they were gloves. We have doctors at ringside. We are well-regulated."

"Isn't it interesting," added McCain, "that someone like Floyd Patterson would say this kind of contest is appalling and repugnant, a former heavyweight champion of the world?"

"Yes, very interesting," chuckled Shamrock, noting the transparency of Patterson's stance. "Why are you laughing, Ken?," asked King.

"I enjoy boxing," Shamrock said. "And I attended a boxing match in Palm Springs not long ago . . . but there's no way around it. In boxing, you have numerous shots to the head—a guy's brain is bouncing around inside of his skull a minimum of fifty or sixty times a fight or more."

McCain's smile was evaporating.

"If the appointed officials who regulate boxing in thirty-six states unanimously agree this is unacceptable, that someone can be maimed . . .," McCain said.

"Then why don't you stop boxing?," Shamrock asked.

McCain remained silent.

"So why don't you stop boxing?," Shamrock asked again.

McCain was no longer smiling at all. "Excuse me for talking while you are interrupting, sir," McCain told Shamrock. "In Las Vegas, where they draw the biggest fights, and everyone knows they are the most respected, they won't touch this with a ten-foot pole. Ask them. Because sooner or later someone is going to get very badly injured," McCain said.

Shamrock could not resist the deepening irony of McCain's argument. "Or maybe, *killed?* You mean *killed?*," Shamrock asked.

McCain smoldered and again retreated to silence. "I guess the point is, people get killed in boxing," King finally said. Shamrock nodded.

After a commercial break, McCain took more heat. Actor and martial artist Robert Conrad, star of "The Wild, Wild West," called in to say he was "surprised, shocked," that McCain was trying to stop the UFC. If martial artists over the age of consent wish to fight on pay-per-view television, Conrad maintained, they should be allowed to do so without the meddling of politicians. "Balance the budget, John," he told McCain.

"What do you have to say to Mr. Conrad, senator?"

"Nothing," snapped McCain. "I hope he will watch one of these fights, as I have watched a part of one, and if he is not appalled, we have nothing in common."

McCain went on to predict that all fifty-one states would ban the UFC, drawing another retort from Shamrock. "How can you say that, senator? It's the politicians who want to ban this, not the people. People have made this one of the most popular pay-per-view events ever. It's the people who elect you; why don't you listen to them?"

McCain, scowling now, ended on a confusing note. "It was mentioned off camera that both Marc and I were at the fight where Bobby Garcia was killed," he said. "It was a very tragic event. I think you could argue that the referee should have stopped the fight before. But there was a referee in the ring and he was doing his best to see that the fighter was not injured."

King seemed taken aback that McCain would cite a boxing fatality bid to vilify the UFC.

"But a man was killed?," King asked.

"Yes," confirmed McCain.

The senator clearly knew or cared little about the UFC's actual safety practices. He had apparently not realized the UFC included a referee and substantial medical supervision. He had apparently not known the event featured professional martial artists, like Shamrock and Dan Severn and Royce Gracie, who had studied their art for years, even decades. And McCain was apparently not aware that the UFC, unlike boxing, allowed fighters to concede defeat at any time— with their dignity intact.

The fatal fight McCain witnessed was held May 6, 1995, in Las Vegas. After enduring eleven rounds of punishment at the hands of Gabriel Ruelas, super-featherweight champion, Garcia collapsed and was rushed to University Medical Center. He lay in a coma for twelve days, until doctors determined he was brain-dead and removed all life-support systems.

Later, in an editorial, the *Los Angeles Times* lambasted Nevada boxing officials for allowing the man to fight, since he had been forced to lose thirty pounds in two months to even qualify for the bout. "Maybe this lopsided fight should never have taken place," suggested the *Times*. "Maybe there was only one way that Garcia should have been allowed anywhere near a ring while Ruelas was fighting: as a spectator."

As he had during most of the discussion on the Larry King show, the senator, in his puzzling reference to the Las Vegas fight, had not revealed the keenest grasp of detail. The young fighter's name was not Bobby Garcia, as McCain said, but Jimmy Garcia, a twenty-three-year-old from Columbia.

Chapter 12

Trouble in Paradise

Isla Verde, Puerto Rico
February 1996

With a graceful spring, he rises instantly from the wave-washed sand, his bronzed muscles stoked with sun and heat. He strides through the sprawling tropical garden court of The Sands, the grand old resort casino of Isla Verde, near San Juan. In the garden are hyacinths and palms and pale-legged, chattering tourists who grow quiet as the man walks past them.

An older couple, visitors from Long Island, are sipping rum and colas at the bar, sunken into the Sands' mammoth free-form pool. "My God, look at this hunk," the woman says. "Now, where did he come from?" The man drawing so many stares moves near. "Probably some dumb weight lifter," her husband says. The bartender is quick to correct them. "No sir," he says. "It is Shamrock. The American fighter. He is very tough. Very good."

It is not merely the man's physique, an impossible inverted pyramid of hardened muscle, that is so striking. It is his walk. A loose, rolling gait, the relaxed movement of a large cat. Shamrock flows away, and the poolside chatter rises again.

A few minutes later, another man appears. He is larger than Shamrock, his 280-pound frame housed in cavernous bib overalls. His face is obscured by a baseball cap, reflective sunglasses, and a Fu Manchu mustache. The man furtively surveys the garden court. He sees the palms, the glistening pool, the beckoning hyacinths, and beyond it, the green phosphorescence of the Caribbean. The man turns and recedes back inside the plushness of The Sands. No one, it seems, noticed Kimo Leopoldo, the "Hawaiian Fighting Legend," the man who slashed at Royce Gracie like a human hurricane, attacked him and maimed him so he could not continue in the tournament of UFC III. Yet today, in this magical setting, Kimo Leopoldo appears to be a man on edge, a man wound very, very tight. There is, perhaps, good reason for Leopoldo to appear anxious. Later this week, in the Ruben Rodriguez Coliseum in nearby Bayamon, he is to face Ken Shamrock in the octagon.

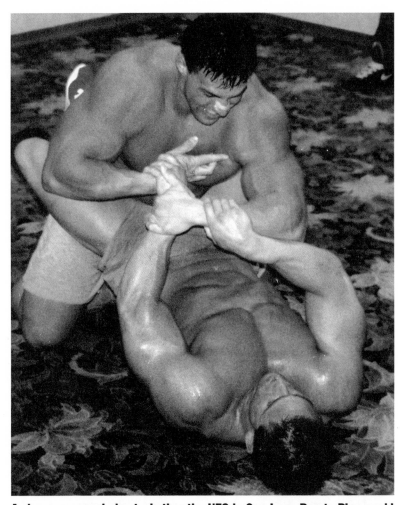

As lawyers argued about whether the UFC in San Juan, Puerto Rico,would go on as planned, Shamrock trained in a make-shift dojo at the Sands hotel and casino with Dan Freeman, a former AAU Mr. California. *(Lions Den photo)*

Judging by the early indications, UFC VIII would be a break-through event for Semaphore Entertainment Group, the company that owns and produces the fight. Perhaps drawn by the trade winds and the beaches, the national press corps has descended to scrutinize the spectacle, condemned by one pundit as "barbaric blood sport." The *LA Times* is ensconced at The Sands. So is the *Philadelphia Inquirer,* even *People* magazine. These are feature writers, in the main, ill-equipped to cover a martial arts event, but directed, groomed, and eager to capture a cultural oddity, a blood-spattered grotesquerie.

Even so, it is an old promoter's adage that bad publicity is usually better than none, so the SEG executives are heartened by the appearance of so many lenses and notebooks.

UFC VIII could be a breakthrough event for Shamrock, as well. His fight against Leopoldo was heralded in a cover story in *Black Belt,* magazine. He has now fought and dominated Gracie, Taktarov, Severn. A victory over Leopoldo would help cement his position as the premier martial artist of his generation.

The welcome media crescendo, though, comes at an indelicate time. There is legal trouble in paradise, a very real chance that Shamrock and Leopoldo may not square off at all; a chance the reportorial pack may not be sated. The government of Puerto Rico, home to one of the world's largest legalized cockfight arenas, and a place where boxing is wildly popular, has decided the UFC is not welcome. Too brutal, contends Eric Labrador, the minister of Sports and Recreation. Too violent, says Gov. Pedro Rossello. No matter that SEG has a valid contract for the rental of Ruben Rodriquez. No matter that the company has invested hundreds of thousands in this event, or has provided extensive written and verbal testimony proving that the UFC is far safer than boxing. The Puerto Rican officials were swayed by missives from the tenacious if ill-informed Senator McCain who told them the event "has no place in a civilized society."

As the issue is being chewed over in U.S. District Court, rumors swirl in the elegant lobby of The Sands, where dowagers dripping with emeralds mix with high-rollers drawn to the craps and poker tables in the adjacent casino. According to the whispered speculation, SEG has hatched back-up plans, just in case the court rules against it. A cargo vessel is supposedly poised to take fighters and technicians to a gymnasium on a nearby island. A fleet of helicopters is being

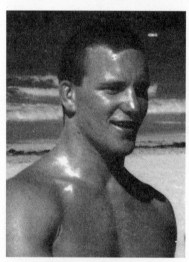

Jerry Bohlander, with a quick smile and friendly manner, seemed almost too nice to compete in the battle zone known as the octagon. He turned out, though, to be a valiant no-holds-barred warrior. *(Lions Den photo)*

assembled to rush the participants to a cruise liner,
where the fight can be staged
at sea.

Shamrock seems oblivi-
ous to the controversy and
idle talk. He has picked up a
slight cold, a gift, he says,
from his wife Tina. Yet the
couple spend pleasant hours
on the beach and poolside
together. The champion is
interviewed by a succession
of reporters, all curious to
explore the background and
psyche of a man anointed the
world's greatest hand-to-
hand warrior. Shamrock even
allows a genial crew from
German public television to

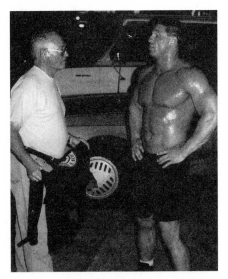

Shamrock gulps air outside the dojo of Michael Cruz in Puerto Rico following a work-out. His dad, Bob, stands by to assist. (Lions Den photo)

shadow him for an entire day, answering unending questions ("What
did you have for breakfast today?") and enduring the hovering sound
boom and video camera. Shamrock does so with good cheer. At the
core an intensely private man, Shamrock shows a surprising and natural ease with reporters, even those whose final work may not be
entirely flattering to him. "I don't mind it," Shamrock says of the
incessant interviewers. "Most of them seem like nice people."

While the Superfight champion is besieged by reporters, another
fighter at The Sands has yet to receive an interview request. Jeremiah
"Jerry" Bohlander is one of Shamrock's fighters, a relatively untested
rookie in the realm of mixed martial arts events. Bohlander, twenty-
one, has turquoise eyes and a gentle manner. He has a quick smile
and makes a point to say, "thank you" and "you are welcome."
Eventually, Bohlander is hoping to win gladiatorial glory with Lion's
Den, but he has a more immediate need, as well: to help support his
mother, badly injured in a car accident, and his two younger sisters.
Bohlander is fighting in the tournament immediately preceding the
Superfight, a tournament billed as "The Davids versus the Goliaths."

"I'm fighting a big guy, a guy six-feet, one-inch and 335 pounds,"
says Bohlander, who is six-feet tall and weighs a little less than 200
pounds. "I'm guessing he is not in the best of shape. I suppose I'll try

to move him around, try him out, then go for a submission hold." His opponent, in fact, is to be Scott "The Pitbull" Ferrozzo of Las Vegas. A former All-America nose guard who bench presses 500 pounds, Ferrozzo has been working extensively with a kickboxing champion to prepare for the UFC. In an interview before he arrived in San Juan, Ferrozzo said he'd been in plenty of fights and had never lost. "You hear how there is always a bigger, tougher guy out there?," Ferrozzo said. "Well, I haven't met him yet."

Bohlander grew up in Montana, wrestled in high school in the Bay Area, and was ready to become an apprentice ironworker when he was transfixed by a tape of UFC III, where Shamrock defeated Leininger and Mitchell. "I liked the way Ken handled himself. He was in really good shape. He fought real aggressively, like a wrestler," Bohlander said. "So I got in touch with Lion's Den. They told me to come over and take some self-defense classes." But Bohlander wasn't required to labor in the self-defense classes for long. During the first session, Shamrock asked if anybody wanted to grapple. Bohlander's arm shot up. He went at it with some of the Lion's Den warriors. He got creamed but showed a valiant fighting spirit. "Bob and Ken asked me afterward if I wanted to try out for the Lion's Den,"

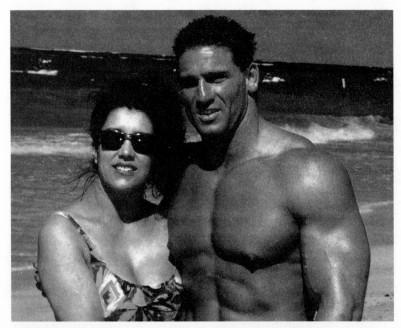

Before his Superfight in Puerto Rico, Shamrock found time to relax on the beach at Isla Verde with his wife, Tina. *(Lions Den photo)*

he said. "I did. And I've been with them ever since." Bohlander's first and only professional fight was in Hawaii, in the Superbrawl Mixed Martial Arts Championship, and he won in less than two minutes. Here in San Juan he has a shot at something larger. Much larger. "Ken feels I can do it. Take the whole thing. He gives me confidence." Still, there is a sweetness about Jerry Bohlander, the young man with turquoise eyes and impeccable manners. A sweetness that prompts some who meet him at The Sands hotel to question whether such a well-mannered young man can prevail in a bloody battle zone known as the octagon. And there is this as well: Jerry Bohlander has been training with Lion's Den just a little more than six months.

It is Wednesday night, forty-eight hours before the fight is to begin, assuming the legal obstacles are cleared aside. Earlier in the day, a U.S. District Court judge, Daniel Dominguez, agreed to take the matter under consideration. Shamrock must continue as if the fight will happen. He has found a dojo where he may spar away from the probing eyes of the reporters and curious competitors at The Sands. The Shamrock entourage leaves the resort for the secret location. On the way, Shamrock is pensive but confident. He sits in the front passenger seat as his father weaves the rental car through the busy San Juan traffic. "This won't be a complicated fight. Kimo is going to come after me like a runaway train. I'll use my submissions. I'll probably take him with a leg submission. Kimo is big and tough, but his technique is not advanced," Shamrock says. In the months since entering his first UFC, Shamrock feels he has honed his own submissions technique to a near-surgical efficiency. "It's not so much about rage, though I need to be aggressive. It is about technique. In the end, it's technique that will decide most fights."

The rental pulls in front of the storefront martial arts studio of Michael Cruz in Levittown, a suburb of San Juan. It is nearly 10:00 P.M., about the time Shamrock will fight Friday night. During the week before a competition, Shamrock always tries to spar at the same time the actual fight is to be held so his body is accustomed to revving up and delivering at the right time. No classes have been held at the dojo tonight, but more than 100 Puerto Ricans, friends and students of Cruz, have gathered. They are hoping for a glimpse of Shamrock. Wearing a black Pancrase bandanna that gives him the look of a buffed-out buccaneer, Shamrock enters the small dojo and begins stretching on the red mat. Against the window, peering through iron bars, are dozens of eyes. Shamrock finishes his stretches, then strips to a pair of black shorts and wrestling shoes. He punches at padded focus gloves held by Masa Funaki, his friend and advisor. Each strike resounds through the small space like a sonic boom. Thwwwwak. Thwwwwak. Thwwwwwwwwwak. Outside, the crowd murmurs. Shamrock goes through his routine, striking with the gloves, practicing takedowns, then moving through the guard and mount positions.

For most of his fights, Shamrock brings in a surrogate for his eventual nemesis. As a stand-in for Kimo, he has recruited Dan Freeman, a former AAU Mr. California bodybuilder and a karate black belt from Modesto, California. When he is not training, Freeman is a radiation therapist at a hospital in Modesto. He weighs 270 pounds, and like Kimo, he is powerful and aggressive. Freeman worked with Shamrock in Lodi at Lion's Den. He continues his impersonation of Kimo in Puerto Rico. Freeman straddles Shamrock, who is on his back. Funaki stands above them. "Ok, Ok," says Funaki, who will serve as both coach and informal referee for this session. Suddenly, Freeman lunges down to control Shamrock with his massive arms. Shamrock bends his leg into the big man's stomach, turns him aside, and escapes. "Yup!" Funaki says approvingly. "Yup. Go. Go more." Freeman and Shamrock work for perhaps fifteen minutes. Shamrock repeatedly escapes, slipping behind Freeman or pretzeling to a position of control or submission. Yet Freeman is a huge, determined opponent, and several times the men's bodies slam hard into the mats and even the walls of the tiny dojo. Each rumble brings more murmurs from the fans collected outside.

After a half hour, the workout is done. Shamrock glistens with sweat. The temperature inside the dojo is nearly 100 degrees, with humidity rivaling that of a sauna. Shamrock walks quickly out of the tiny dojo into the night. He circles in the parking lot, hands on hips, gulping air until his body is finally cool enough to pull back on his shirt and bandanna. But the visit is not over. Word has quickly spread that Shamrock is training here, in the martial arts studio of Michael Cruz, in a working-class neighborhood. The crowd has grown. Everyone, it seems, wants to connect with the big man who looks like a pirate. "I see him fight on TV," says a man with a graying mustache, waiting to meet the fighter. "I like his style. I like his heart." Freeman, spent from the sparring, uses a towel to absorb the rivers of sweat pouring out of his gigantic chest. "Ken is so quick, so deceptive, so smart," Freeman says. "He's always thinking, thinking ahead. Just when you think you have him, boom, he's out and on top of you."

In front of the dojo, Shamrock poses for dozens of photos, signs countless autographs, shakes hand after hand. He lingers for more than an hour, until each request has been satisfied.

On Thursday, Shamrock rises late and relaxes. There will be no
more interviews. With the fight just one day way, Shamrock must now
begin to muster body and soul for the battle ahead. Over a lunch of
grilled tuna and rice with salad in a patio restaurant at The Sands,
Shamrock talks quietly about Kimo Leopoldo. "If he hits me, he could
hurt me. Royce couldn't hurt me. Kimo could. So I have to get close
to him, control him. It will not be a long fight," he says. "Kimo does-
n't want a long fight. And I don't need one to do what I need to do."
Talk at the table, shared by Shamrock and several of his friends and
supporters, drifts to various tourist spots in Puerto Rico. Shamrock's
eyes, pools of green and silver, gaze out over the pool, across the
palms and lacy bamboo forest, to the sparking jade of the Caribbean.
"Have you been to Old San Juan?," a friend asks him. Shamrock does
not answer. He is no longer in a garden cafe enjoying grilled tuna with
friends. His mind has disengaged. It has raced to an octagon enclosed
by black mesh. Shamrock sees himself inside the fighting pit across
from a man with a Fu Manchu beard and a tattoo of the name "Jesus"
etched into his chest.

And he sees a fight unfold, furious and quick.

Chapter 13

Bullfight

Bayamon, Puerto Rico
February 8, 1996

T he fight, as you have probably heard, is on," announces Art
Davie. "We are delighted to be here in Puerto Rico. We will
be back." There is a ripple of applause from the assemblage
of men wearing sweat suits and in-your-face expressions. It is
Thursday night, time for the manager and fighter meeting, held in the
grand ballroom at The Sands.

Earlier in the day, Judge Dominquez ruled the government could
not block the UFC because it had no regulations governing such
fights. He also found that the financial blow to SEG should the UFC
be stopped would be far greater than the harm to the government if
the event proceeded. Davie, clearly pleased, gestures with an unlit
cigar the size of a salami as he stands before the group of perhaps
fifty. "It's a pleasure to welcome you all. Each of you is steeped in
your art. Please don't listen to the press or the politicians. They simply do not know what they are talking about." The roomful of men,
most with chests and biceps pumped big by years of training, provides another trickle of applause. In the UFC's brief history, the managers' meeting has become one of the rituals of the event. It is a time
to go through the rules, meet the event's big wheels, maybe sling a
stare or two at the competition. Davie finishes and the floor is taken
over by John McCarthy, the towering Los Angeles cop who is the
event's referee.

McCarthy teaches defensive tactics to officers and has a background in martial arts himself. Dressed in a white polo shirt and black
pants, he is plain-spoken, blunt, purposeful. "Let's go over some
expectations," he says. "First, cut the nails. This isn't a girl's cat fight.
If you don't trim 'em way down, I'll have to pull out my clippers and
trim 'em down for you while three million people watch us."
McCarthy goes over acceptable clothing: t-shirts, tank tops, gis. "You
must have shorts with a drawstring. And wear a pair of undershorts
below those shorts. You don't want to be exposed on live TV." The

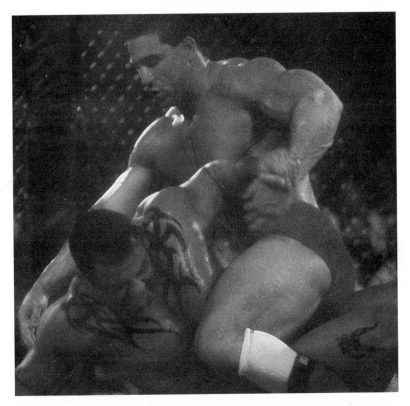

Shamrock, positioned behind Kimo Leopoldo, chose not to strike or choke him during his Superfight in Puerto Rico. Shamrock was determined to use a leg submission against his Superfight opponent. *(SEG photo)*

fighters must all wear steel cups and mouthpieces. No rings or earrings are allowed. No heavy greases or lotions are allowed, either. "If it looks wet, it will be rubbed off." McCarthy pauses and asks for questions. No one speaks up. "Okay, let's go over the rules. There aren't many. No eye-gouging. Keep your hands away from the eyes. No biting. No throat strikes. No fish-hooking." One manager raises his hand and asks what that is. "It's jamming your finger into your opponent's mouth and trying to tear his cheek out," explains another manager. McCarthy continues. "If you are taking undue punishment, I will stop a fight. If your corner throws in a towel, I will stop a fight. If you are seriously hurt or knocked out, I will stop it. Any other questions?" The room is silent. "Oh, there is one more rule," he says. "Don't hit the referee. He hits back."

By virtue of his status and experience, Shamrock is not required to attend the manager's meeting. But he is nearby, in meeting room

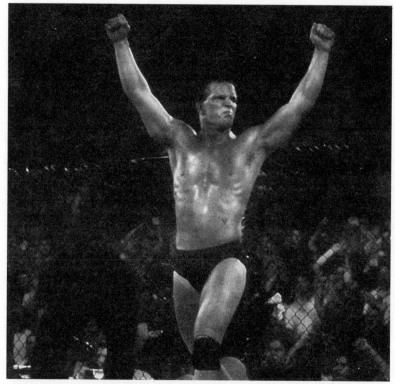

Jerry Bohlander showed tremendous patience in his fight with Scott Ferrozzo (background) eventually choking him out and becoming the youngest UFC winner in the history of the event. *(SEG photo)*

one at the Sands, in a salon with thick brocaded carpet where the watercolor paintings of palms and sailboats have been removed from the walls. For tonight, this final night before the Superfight, this conference room, usually occupied by business types with briefcases, has become a dojo, a sparring space. Lion's Den, Isla Verde.

"Inside, inside. Hands inside," Funaki tells Shamrock, as he charges at Freeman. Shamrock has been clenching Freeman around the arms, instead of knifing his hands between his arms and ribcage, the more strategic position. Shamrock rushes Freeman again, deftly slipping his arms around his ribcage like a linebacker ready to demolish a tailback. "Yup. Good," Funaki says. "Very good. Take short break." Masa Funaki is the closest thing Shamrock has to a coach. He helped teach submissions to Shamrock in Japan and is regarded as one of the most technically proficient martial artists in the world. Now thirty-two, Funaki has been a submissions fighter since age fifteen. He has also studied karate, muay Thai, and ju-jitsu.

Funaki fights in the Pancrase arena, but he is also one of its founders and top executives. He has a nimble and penetrating mind and has pondered the nearly infinite ways the human body may be subtly manipulated and controlled. "He could go into the octagon and take anybody," says Frank Shamrock. "Anybody, that is, except Ken."

Funaki leans against the wallpaper of the salon, taking a sip of water from a battle. Asked how he thinks the Superfight will go, he does not hesitate. "Ken be like steering the cow," he says. A puzzled reporter looks at a Japanese photographer, who confers with Funaki. The photographer, who speaks very good English, offers a translation. "Funaki says Ken will be the bullfighter. Kimo will be the bull." Funaki continues, saying Shamrock need not focus much on Kimo. Shamrock, he says, must focus on Shamrock. "In fighting, it is not other person. It is self," he said. "Control self, you have a good chance of winning. Not control self, not so good a chance of winning." Funaki is nothing if not the personification of control. He has a handsome face that seldom reveals a trace of emotion. After the short break, Funaki himself spars with Bohlander. At one point, Bohlander shoves Funaki onto his back against a wall, then manages to drive an elbow across his neck. Funaki's position seems both painful and untenable. But his eyes are dark and impassive, the eyes of a man who could be watching a sparrow dance across the sky. Suddenly, he whips a leg over Bohlander's back, slides his head under Bohlander's elbow, and slips behind him to a position that could quickly lead to Bohlander being choked out. The sequence happens in perhaps three seconds. "Yup. Okay. Okay," Funaki tells Bohlander. "You ready now."

It is Friday, February 16. Fight day. Shamrock is in no hurry to rise. He sleeps until 11:00 A.M. Then he orders in a breakfast of steak, eggs, potatoes, toast, rice, and salad. Shamrock will eat twice more this day, sandwiches and pizza and more salad. It is fuel for battle, fuel that will take most of the day to ingest and perhaps ten minutes to burn up in frenetic combat.

About the time Shamrock finishes his steak and eggs in his suite, a bus loaded with reporters and fighters and UFC workers pulls away from The Sands. The bus wends through San Juan to the coliseum for a walk-through of the venue and the octagon. Shamrock has been through several walk-throughs and skips this one. Among those on board the bus is Leon Tabbs, cut man, trainer, and raconteur. A former Air Force medic, Tabbs is flown to each UFC from his home in Philadelphia for one reason: he can stop the flow of blood better than anyone outside an operating room. He carries a bag immaculately packed with various potions that can constrict vessels, cause blood to coagulate, slow the reddish oozing from a well-struck brow or nose or chin. Tabbs was a boxer, then a manager. But he quickly discovered it made sense to learn something of the cutman's art. "It cost money to hire a cut man," he said. "In those days, we didn't make a lot of money. So if I was managing a fighter, I was his cut man, too." Tabbs eventually stopped managing boxers altogether and concentrated on tending to their wounds. He was worked with Evander Holyfield and Jerry Martin, among others. Asked how Shamrock would do against a boxer, Tabbs savors the thought like a connoisseur tasting a fine wine. "Oh, that would be interesting," he says, after a few seconds. "Shamrock is in amazing condition. I had to examine all the fighters, and I examined Ken. The man is like a rock. I mean, he's *hard.* He's also a tough guy who really knows how to grapple. A boxer would have to get some good shots in fast to have a chance. Otherwise, Shamrock would take him to the ground and it would be over," Tabbs says.

Leon Tabbs thinks for a moment more, rubs his chin thoughtfully, and offers a final comment. "Ken Shamrock, when you get down to it, would kick Mike Tyson's butt."

At 4:00 P.M., in his suite at The Sands, Ken Shamrock is watching a movie. It is *Deadman Walking,* about a condemned man facing the ultimate punishment. On the day of the fight, there is no work-out, although there will be a strenuous warm-up later at the coliseum in Bayamon. In the hours before he must dress and leave the hotel, Shamrock often watches movies. Action or drama, the movies allow him to relax. Some, like *Deadman Walking,* or *Glory,* about African-American soldiers facing horrible odds in a Civil War battle, provide a sobering perspective. "If people have faced execution or a battle they are probably going to die fighting, it makes what I do look pretty reasonable," he says. From time to time, his mind drifts to the fight, to Kimo. But mostly, his mind adheres to the words and images on the glowing screen before him.

Ken Shamrock firmly believes that ninety-percent or more of a fight is in the preparation. The preparation is done.

● ● ●

As a mob of his fellow citizens howl with satisfaction, Thomas Ramirez, all 410 pounds of him, stumbles backward and drops like a side of beef to the canvas. Like images of cherries in a slot machine, his eyes roll back into his head. Then, his brain circuitry re-connecting, he blinks, the eyes click back into position, and the big man from Bayamon slowly realizes that he is lying on his back on a canvas ring in front of an audience that approaches the population of Puerto Rico. In the first bout of UFC XIII, Ramirez has been knocked senseless by a firefighter named Don Frye from Bizbee, Arizona. The demolition lasted less than ten seconds. It is 10:15 P.M.

The show has begun.

It is a steamy tropical night in Bayamon and the crowd of 8,000 has been downing oceans of Budweiser and piña coladas to loosen up and cool off. The Ruben Rodriguez coliseum, for whatever reason, has no air conditioning. It is moist as a swamp. Many of the spectators, some of whom entered the venue two hours before the first bout, are now soused and drenched with sweat. Frye's efficient victory over the massive Ramirez was not the first contest of the night; security officers have broken up a half-dozen drunken skirmishes, some including the use of folding metal chairs as bludgeons.

The arena has no locker rooms. Curtains have been erected to form a series of cubicles and these cramped spaces are where the fighters warm-up before their bouts. There is one exception. Shamrock, given his due as reigning Superfight royalty, is ensconced in a large rest room. With him are his father, several of the Lion's Den fighters, and Jerry Bohlander. Only a few minutes after the Frye-Ramirez bout, an SEG worker raps on the door. "Bohlander up next," he says. Bohlander, wearing black Speedo shorts and black knee pads, marches with Frank Shamrock toward the center of the arena, to the black enclosure where he will do battle.

Bohlander's opponent, Scott Ferrozzo, is already there. He has removed a smock scrawled with the words, "FEAR ME," exposing 330 pounds of flesh. But unlike the flabby Ramirez, Ferrozzo, thirty-one, is solid, his upper body a monolith of sinew and muscle. And Ferrozzo's eyes are dark and steady. He appears as immovable as Everest.

At McCarthy's signal, the fighters converge. The fight will have a ten-minute time limit. Like the former nose guard he is, Ferrozzo tackles Bohlander and manages to hurl him into the chain-link of the octagon. With all of his might and weight, he presses Bohlander against the fence, as if trying to press a slab of cheese through a grater. Bohlander, lean and compact, seems to be nearly consumed by Ferrozzo. Yet he manages to free one fist and starts smacking Ferrozzo's neck, face, and ears. Bohlander has launched a modest but methodical offense, akin to a woodpecker taking chunks out of a pine.

More important, in these first moments, the UFC rookie has not panicked under the stifling bulk of his adversary. "Look at Bohlander," says Jeff Blatnick, a UFC commentator. "Look at how poised he is." After almost seven minutes of pecking away, Bohlander draws a stream of crimson from Berrozzo's forehead. McCarthy stops the fight and Tabbs and the ring physicians quickly review the cut and deem it minor. The bout continues, but Ferrozzo again seizes Bohlander and bulldozes him into the fence. Blatnick states what has become clear: "Ferrozzo doesn't know what to do next." The huge fighter is also growing weary. With less than a minute to go, Ferrozzo senses he must do something, anything, to break the stalemate. He suddenly releases, rocks backward, and pulls Bohlander to the canvas, hoping to squash or strike him. Bohlander is too quick. He rolls out of Ferrozzo's grasp, and coils an arm around Ferrozzo's neck. Ferrozzo rears like a wounded grizzly, but Bohlander will not let go. With Bohlander glued to his neck, Ferrozzo surges again toward the familiar terrain of the chain link. He slams Bohlander against the fence but cannot shake him off. Steadily, the choke sinks into the airways and arteries within the enormous neck of Scott Ferrozzo. Finally, the wounded bear can take no more. Ferrozzo slumps to the canvas and taps out.

In the bathroom that is Shamrock's staging area, the Lion's Den crew goes ballistic as Bohlander enters. He is hugged and slapped and embraced by a chorus of congratulations. Then Shamrock's voice booms out. "Everybody quiet," he says. "Quiet now. Jerry won and that's great. But he has another fight. He's not done yet." Bohlander sits down and towels himself off. He tries to cool, relax, and catch his breath, recover from the siege he has just endured. But there is scant time. He must fight again soon, and the fickle nature of tournament fighting has not been kind. Not kind at all.

In ten minutes, the door is rapped again, and again Bohlander is summoned. He faces Gary Goodridge, a 260-pound boxer and practitioner of a Korean martial art, kuk sool won, which stresses strikes and kicks. In his preliminary bout, Goodridge trapped former wrestler Paul Herrera and stretched him out like a pig on a spit. Herrera, legs clamped between Goodridge's knees, his arm trapped below Goodridge, could not budge. What happened next alarmed SEG executives, for it was perhaps the most terrifying episode in the history of the event. Goodridge slammed his elbow into Herrera's jaw. The first blow, delivered with the apparent force of a baseball bat, knocked Herrera out cold. Goodridge, electric with adrenaline and unaware

Herrera was out, continued the barrage. His powerful elbow dropped into Herrera's face and jaw again. And again. And again. And again. Herrera's entire body shook from the power of the blows. McCarthy scrambled to halt the beating. Before he did, in less than four seconds, Goodridge had slammed his elbow eight times into the motionless face and skull of Paul Herrera. It took a long minute before Herrera was roused from his slumber, and he later spent the night at a hospital for treatment of a concussion and broken jaw. (Producers of the UFC, usually eager to highlight dramatic kicks and strikes, instantly realized the unseemly excess of the attack. There was not a single replay of the Goodridge victory.)

The ferocity of Goodridge's win is of little matter to Bohlander. After sparring for many weeks with Shamrock, Bohlander will not be intimidated. But the bout against the inspired Ferrozzo has winded him, and the humidity and heat of the arena has conspired to thwart his recovery. After ten grueling minutes against a much larger man, he faces another much larger man whose fight lasted less than nine seconds. Still, Bohlander fights gamely. For a brief time, he even mounts Goodridge and appears ready to finish him off with a series of blows to the head. But Bohlander's arms have turned rubbery. The blows do not find their mark. Goodridge easily fends them off, then manages to rear up, flip Bohlander to the mat, and push him against the fence. Goodridge, with a superior reach, stands above Bohlander and bombs him with massive fists. Mindful of the mayhem Goodridge wreaked on Herrera, McCarthy swiftly steps in and stops the fight after five minutes and thirty-three seconds. It is the arm of Goodridge that is hoisted in victory. But it is Bohlander who has proven his mettle. Tonight the sweet-natured kid from Livermore has become the youngest fighter to claim a victory in the octagon.

Kimo Leopoldo is waiting now, standing with one leg slightly in front of the other. He has entered the arena with head bowed, below a cryptic sign with a crucifix and the message: "If I Am Okay And You Are Okay, Then How Do You Explain This?" As he stands on the grey-blue canvas of the octagon, there seems none of the spark, the fury, that propelled his assault on Royce Gracie. Kimo, twenty-eight, was a cipher before that bout, and he has remained a cipher since. During interviews, he has acknowledged a battle with addictive drugs, from mushrooms to steroids to pot. He has talked of finding God, of beating his addictions, of using the octagon as a pulpit of sorts. "Preaching the word of the Lord is what it's about, and fighting is how I can do it."

Ken Shamrock, in red Speedo shorts, is about thirty feet from Leopoldo now. He bounces easily, lightly. He is loose and relaxed. Shamrock's eyes are expressionless and steady as lasers. It is already playing in his head, a vision of the fight, the moves, the ending. He peers into the eyes of Kimo Leopoldo and sees uncertainty. Kimo blinks. "Alright, let's get it on," McCarthy says. Kimo charges at Shamrock and flings a wild kick at him. Shamrock responds with a solid right smash to the face, and the fighters collapse in a jumble of writhing limbs. The crowd of sweat-soaked Puerto Ricans scream their approval. Shamrock holds Leopoldo down and throws quick, stinging punches to his ribs. Kimo manages a headbutt, then dislodges Shamrock. Shamrock, whirling behind the Hawaiian, has a chance, a clear opening to land a crushing strike to the neck or head. He does not strike. The tape playing in Shamrock's mind shows a submission hold, not a finishing flurry of strikes. Shamrock lunges for Leopoldo's leg but it is wet and slick as a big mackerel. He tries again, this time capturing the slippery limb and jamming it between his own legs. Leopoldo tries to shake Shamrock off, then tries to roll him off. He can do neither. Shamrock has claimed the leg as his own, and now he controls it in a knee bar. Swiftly, Shamrock wrenches the limb, straining the cartilage and ligaments in Leopoldo's knee to the bursting point. It is hopeless. Leopoldo can either tap the canvas or watch his knee explode before his eyes. He desperately slams his hand down three times.

Ken Shamrock remains the Superfight champion of the UFC.

Shamrock and Leopoldo rise and embrace in the center of the ring. "Great fight," Leopoldo says. "It was a great fight," answers Shamrock. "God bless you."

At the post-fight party in the main ballroom at The Sands, there is a buffet of fajitas and rice and shrimp. The fighters and managers and their well-wishers crowd around the bars set up on either end of the huge room, eager to celebrate, eager to wash away the stress of the previous week and the tension of the evening's battles. Some of the attendees are on the dance floor, moving to a tape-recorded version of "Start Me Up," by the Rolling Stones.

For Jerry Bohlander, it has been a testing night, but a good one. He is $5,000 richer, he has a UFC victory to his credit, and he is a young man with a bright future in the tough but glamorous world of no-holds-barred fighting. Even with a nasty mouse rising over his right eye, his wholesome, All-America good looks remain. He is repeatedly asked to pose for photos with party-goers. Among those posing with Bohlander are two of the octagon girls, the shapely women in bikinis who circle the fighting pit before each contest holding signs listing each man's martial art. The octagon girls are in evening gowns now, looking hot and glittery. Jerry Bohlander is smiling broadly as the flash goes off.

Shamrock holds court at a victory table that includes his father, wife, Funaki, and Masami Ozaki, the president of Pancrase. The fight unfolded much as he planned, he said. "No surprises," he tells friends. Funaki agrees. "Like we thought. Ken fight the bull," he says. Shamrock wears slacks, a vest and gold chain, a light, cool ensemble that reveals his monster chest and biceps. Shamrock sips wine, scribbles autographs, shakes dozens of hands. This is his moment, a luminous one. He has won more than $50,000 tonight, he remains the undisputed Superfight champion of the UFC and continues to be one of the most heralded martial arts figures in the country. (A *People* magazine article published the next week says Shamrock, "is the UFC's Golden Boy, blond and handsome." The writer apparently did not see the photo accompanying the article revealing a distinctly dark-haired Ken Shamrock.)

Busy talking at his table, Shamrock does not notice a television not far away in a corner of the banquet room. A videotape of UFC VIII is being played. The tape shows Shamrock's Superfight triumph over Leopoldo. Then the tape shows the mustachioed face of Dan Severn, sitting at ringside in the Ruben Rodriquez Coluseum. It has already been announced that Shamrock, having retained his belt, will square off in a rematch against Severn in Detroit's Cobo Arena.

"Shamrock will be coming to my home state this time," Severn says. "He'll be coming to my house. He'll be violating my territory. It will be different this time."

Chapter 14

Blood Brothers

Lodi
May 2, 1996

Shamrock pulls up outside of a Lodi bar and grill in his Dodge pick-up truck, the huge black beast with the ten-cylinder Viper engine. He has finished an evening work-out and has agreed to meet two old friends for a beer. Shamrock has never been a heavy drinker and now, as a busy young father, he partakes even more sparingly. Yet his schedule has kept him busy of late, so busy he has not had much time with family, let alone friends. So tonight is a rare chance to reconnect with some buddies.

As Shamrock and his friends talk at the bar, patrons begin noticing the fighter, wearing a black Lion's Den T-shirt, nylon sweat pants, and three days worth of beard stubble. Just two years ago, Shamrock could go anywhere in Lodi without being recognized. Now, almost everywhere he goes, people stop and stare or point or even venture up close to ask for an autograph from the fighter with the Adonis build.

A man with beefy forearms and orange hair has noticed Shamrock in the bar. The man is sitting alone at a small table littered with cigarette butts and empty beer mugs. The man squashes a Camel and rises to his feet. He is well over six feet tall, wearing cowboy boots and a tank top. He is lumbering toward Shamrock.

The fighter, his natural antennae twitching, tilts his head and sees the big man moving toward him.

There was a time when the next few minutes would include an explosion of fists and perhaps a 911 call for an ambulance. But with some age and the accumulation of creature comforts, Shamrock is learning to tame the rage. He must control it, or risk losing it all. A hand broken in a bar brawl could put him out of the next fight, could cost him dearly, his family dearly. A nasty headline, and the would-be movie action star may get nothing but Hollywood's crumbs.

The big lumbering redhead is among a defective class of men who now, from time to time, challenge Shamrock's self-control. During the party following UFC VI, after Shamrock had taken out Severn, the

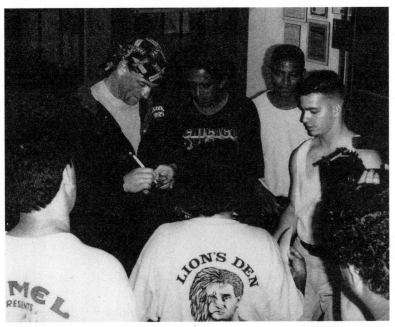

With his UFC success, Shamrock gained celebrity status. But his fame sometimes drew misguided sorts wanting to test the person known as the world's most dangerous man. *(Lions Den photo)*

bad boy of no-holds-barred fighting, Tank Abbott, the feral pit fighter from Long Beach, approached Shamrock and leaned over to his ear. "Great fight," Abbott offered. "You were pretty tough out there."

Shamrock thanked him. "But you know what?," Abbot continued. "I'm awful tough, too. In fact, I think I'm tough enough to kick your ass."

The bluster failed to ignite Shamrock.

"Well, who knows, Tank," he replied. "Maybe you could."

Abbott, apparently satisfied, swaggered away.

Now the man in cowboy boots has sidled up and offered his hand. "Hey, aren't you Ken Shamrock, the ultimate fighter?" the redhead says, his words morphed by an intemperate ingestion of Coors. Shamrock shakes the fellow's hand and confirms his status as the reigning hand-to-hand warrior in the country. The man praises Shamrock for a few minutes, then starts bragging about his own fighting prowess. He's won a few bar fights in his time, he says. "I stay in pretty good shape, too. I can still bench press 300," he says. Shamrock looks into the man's eyes and sees something switch on, something he doesn't like, something he often saw when he patrolled saloons as a bouncer. "Hey, buddy, let me buy you a beer," Shamrock says, slapping cash on the bar. The man continues, "You know what, Shamrock? You don't look so damn mean," the man in cowboy boots says. "I bet I could take you. I'll bet I could take you right here, right now." Shamrock feels a jolt of the anger, the old anger, welling to the surface. It would be so easy, so satisfying, to allow the man to swing, and then crush him. But Shamrock holds steady. "You never know," Shamrock says, sliding a fresh Coors in front of the deluded man. "Nice meeting you. I gotta run."

Shamrock shakes hands with his friends and departs. Then the world's most accomplished fighter and a man steadily gaining restraint and maturity drives home to a quiet subdivision, where his wife and three children are already asleep.

Ken Shamrock's adoptive father, Bob, began the process of making his son whole, a process that continued with Ken's marriage to Tina. But Shamrock's children have sharply accelerated that process. They have allowed him to grow far beyond the man he once was.

Through both his earnings as a professional athlete and his desire to change, he has given his sons a peaceful and secure boyhood he never enjoyed himself. Along the way, he has experienced some of the joys he never knew growing up in Georgia and Napa. "At one of the boy's birthday parties, we all had those goofy, pointy hats," Tina recalls. "At the end of the party, there was only one person, adult or child, who was still wearing his funny little hat. That was Ken."

Shamrock sometimes looks at his three sons, Ryan, Connor, and Sean, and thinks of the three boys in Savannah, the three boys hustling on the streets for table scraps and dignity. Bonded by blood and the adversity they shared, those boys, those three brothers have remained close as adults. All three ended up roaming, running away, thieving, experimenting with drugs. All three were processed through juvenile hall and sent to various group or foster homes.

Richie Kilpatrick, the oldest of the brothers, had various brushes with the law during his youth for fighting and stealing and using drugs. In his teens, he visited his brother, Ken, in Susanville, and wound up taking a swing at a cop who was trying to break up a party. He was hauled to jail and was released only after Bob Shamrock vouched for him. He was ordered not to step foot in Susanville again. Richie worked construction and factory jobs in California and Texas and Mississippi and for several years battled an addiction to methamphetamine, commonly called speed. He has been drug-free for nearly three years with the help of his love, Debbie, with whom he has a child.

Robbie, the second oldest of the three, had perhaps the roughest

time. He did a stint in a California Youth Authority lock-up for burglary and drug possession. At the age of eighteen, he was sentenced
to Jamestown Conservation Camp, a state prison, for armed robbery.
He was, he recalls, one of the youngest persons from Napa ever sentenced to state prison. "I asked for it. I thought it would be a shorter
sentence," he said. It ended up being extended after Kilpatrick was
stabbed during a fight in the prison's weight room. He was later transferred to Folsom State Prison, then did time in solitary at Jamestown
before finishing his term at the California Men's Colony in San Luis
Obispo. He worked at various jobs, and even assisted his younger
brother as a bouncer at Doc's Skyroom in Redding for a time. He
wound up serving another term in state prison though, doing time at
Pelican Bay near Eureka on a drug-related offense. Robbie, strong
and well-built, has worked out with Shamrock's fighters and hopes
one day to enter a reality combat tournament himself.

Shamrock knows he was spared some of the troubles suffered by
his brothers only because he met a man named Bob Shamrock in the
mountain town of Susanville. "If I hadn't gone to Susanville, hadn't
met Bob, I would be hooked on drugs now, or in prison, or dead,"
Shamrock said.

Through their misfortunes and misadventures, the three brothers
never lost touch. Ken Shamrock visited Robbie in prison, even sent
him care packages with vitamins and nutritional supplements. With
Robbie out of prison, Shamrock, blessed with a wife and family and a
comfortable home, invites his brothers over for barbecues and birthday and holiday celebrations. "All the stuff we've been through," said
Richie Kilpatrick, "it seems it has only brought us closer."

At Shamrock's invitation, Richie and his companion Debbie flew
to Puerto Rico and attended Shamrock's fight in Bayamon against
Kimo Leopoldo.

Also at Shamrock's invitation, Robbie will soon fly to Detroit to
watch UFC IX, featuring Shamrock's rematch against Severn. It is a fight
that only weeks ago Shamrock seemed relatively unconcerned about.

That is changing, though. Changing rapidly.

● ● ●

The Lion's Den
May 4, 1996
Shamrock has continued his tradition of bringing in fighters to impersonate his upcoming opponents. The man chosen to play Dan Severn

is Mike Radnov, a 260-pound former wrestler and football player at the University Nebraska. Radnov is a personal trainer in Dallas. Shamrock, based on the few sparring sessions he has had with Radnov, believes Radnov is as big as Severn, probably stronger, definitely quicker.

The two are in the fighting ring at the Lion's Den, both working fast and hard, both sweating heavily. Shamrock fires toward Radnov, clinches, takes him down. The concrete walls of Lion's Den seem to quiver as the big men slam to the floor of the ring. "Alright, Mike. Good. Good. Let's just do another couple of minutes," Shamrock says. Shamrock shoots on Radnov and the two drop. Shamrock grasps Radnov's leg and tries to straighten it and apply a kneebar. But Radnov shakes the leg free for a split-second, and the shin slams into Shamrock's nose. Shamrock regains control of the leg and forces Radnov to tap out. Then he rises and holds his reddened nose. "Damn. It's busted," he says. Shamrock's nose has been broken before. It is, on the scale of relative impairment, not a serious injury. Yet it is a telling one.

Later, holding a towel moistened with cold water under his nose, Shamrock concedes he is not on schedule for the fight with Severn. The acting in *Champions,* the T-ball coaching chores, the demands for interviews and photo spreads, have all taken precious time away from his training.

"I'm not slow. I'm not fat," Shamrock says, pinching the towel around his nostrils. "But there are a lot of ways to be out of shape. My stamina is not where it should be. My timing is not where it should be. My head is not where it should be. I still have a lot of work to do."

Shamrock pulls the towel away. It is now spackled with crimson, evidence that Shamrock's timing is not what it might be.

It is thirteen days until the fight in Cobo Arena.

Chapter 15

Superfight

Cobo Arena
Detroit
May 17 1996

In no-holds-barred contests, fighters strive for a single position above all others. It is called the mount. The fighter who has mounted his opponent has straddled him and climbed squarely onto his chest. There, he looms above his opponent, enjoying every

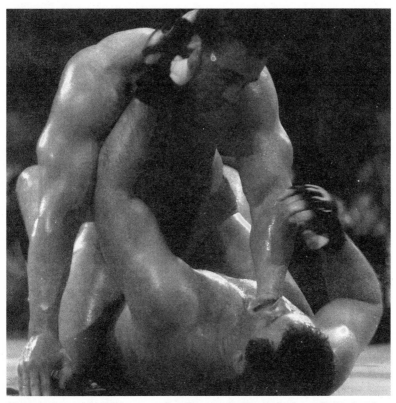

Shamrock succeeded in mounting Severn during their Superfight, but he refused to strike his opponent, passing up a key tactical advantage.
(Calixtro Romias photo)

advantage of reach and leverage and gravity. Fighters who have achieved the mount typically bombard their opponents with strikes to the face and head, forcing a quick surrender. The unfortunate fighter who ends up being mounted can try to muster a defense by raising his hands to protect the fragile bones and tissue of his face. He can attempt to roll out of the mount and risk exposing his back and neck and inviting a rear choke. Or he can simply avoid the inevitable physical punishment and tap out.

At 11:21 P.M., Michigan time, in the center of Cobo Arena, below the hot white television lights, in front of a hostile capacity crowd whistling and screaming its disdain for him, and in front of four-million pay-per-view customers, Ken Shamrock, the Superfight champion of the world, has mounted Dan Severn.

He grinds his muscular bulk into Severn, pins him as surely as a fallen barn rafter. The fight, so far a cautious and disappointing waltz, appears to be nearing a sudden end. "Go ahead, Shamrock," screams a Detroit fan, weary of the defensive shuffle that has defined the fight so far. "Finish the bum off."

Shamrock teaches his Lion's Den students that in most fights there is a turning point, a moment of opportunity. When this moment emerges, it must be seized without hesitation, without restraint. Such a moment has emerged here and now, in Cobo Arena, as Shamrock straddles his fallen opponent. Yet Shamrock's hand does not coil into a hardened fist, a finishing weapon.

For reasons known to few beyond his father and wife and Lion's Den brethren, Shamrock will not strike Severn's face tonight with a closed fist.

• • •

It is the afternoon before the Ultimate Fighting Championship IX. Ken, Tina, and Bob Shamrock have driven in a rented Lincoln to Canada, to The Penalty Box in Windsor. There, they are seated at a long banquet table nearly groaning under the weight of platters piled high with prime rib and chicken breasts and salmon steaks. Also at the table are Robert Meyrowitz and Don Frye, the fighter who won the UFC tournament in Puerto Rico. The Penalty Box is an old-fashioned sports bar and grill that features good, unadorned food, plenty of it, and a variety of draft beer to wash it all down with. Photos of Gordie Howe and Joe Louis stare down from the walls. It is not the usual late afternoon crowd, though: the tables are filled

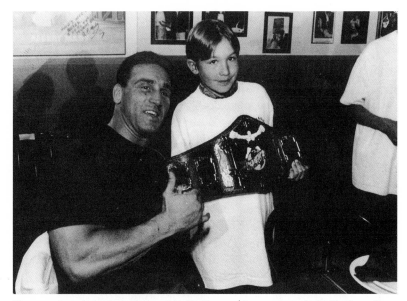

Shamrock makes donations of both time and money on behalf of youth. Here he helps a boy heft his Superfight belt during an appearance for the Windsor Boys and Girls Club before the Superfight in Detroit. (Calixtro Romias photo)

with chattering kids, most wearing T-shirts that say, "Windsor Boys and Girls Club."

Between mouthfuls of rigatoni and salmon, Shamrock signs autographs and poses for photos with the children. The boys and girls seem awed by the man with the raptorial eyes and the bulging chest, who nevertheless, as each approaches, is quick to smile and take their hand in his. "We've had other pro athletes meet the kids, but I prefer these UFC fighters," says Nick Marentette, executive director of the Boys and Girls Club of Windsor. "They are the most down to earth. They don't charge for autographs. They are human." (Among the board members for the youth club is Dave Beneteau, a UFC veteran, a paramedic in Windsor and one of the finest role models to emerge from the event. Unfortunately, he will be blocked from competing in UFC IX, as scheduled, because of a broken hand.)

When the supper is finished, Meyrowitz makes a short speech and donates a check to the club. Then Ken Shamrock moves to the microphone and offers a few words of encouragement to the kids, telling them they will have opportunities in their lives, they will have a chance to make a difference. "Don't give up, even if you have hardships or tough times. Don't give up on your dreams," he says. On behalf of the Shamrocks and Lion's Den, he donates a check to the club as well.

At each of the Superfights, the Shamrocks donate money to a local group serving youngsters, typically a Boys and Girls Club or a YMCA. Shamrock prefers the donations be made quietly, without media present. Shamrock was without hope himself, or nearly so, as a youngster. Now, as a professional athlete, he wants to reach out to other kids and show them it can be done: they can become somebody.

"We are not telling kids they should become professional athletes or fighters," says Bob Shamrock, now guiding the Lincoln back to Detroit. "We're telling them to keep working, to keep striving, to follow their dreams, whether that means graduating from high school or working to be teacher or a doctor."

In Puerto Rico, on the day before the Superfight with Kimo, the Shamrocks discovered an orphanage in the hills above San Juan. With no reporters invited, the Shamrocks, joined by a few UFC officials, ventured on a winding, unpaved road to the orphanage. It was a sparse compound, with some children actually living in former cargo containers. One of the boys, standing well back, is known among social workers as a "cutter," a child who self-mutilates by slicing at himself. After Shamrock presented a check to the man who runs the orphanage, a pick-up basketball game was organized. Shamrock would choose one child to be one his team and Gerry Harris, a UFC fighter who stands six-foot, eight-inches, would chose another child for his team. Shamrock's eyes peered through the forest of young hands stretched high in hopes of being the fighter's teammate. But his eyes focused on a boy standing by himself, well behind the others. "How about you? Back there. Come on up." It was the boy with the pinkish lines running across his hands and arms. All of the children and UFC people circled around the dusty basketball court. The light-hearted contest progressed with the boy failing to score a point. Then Shamrock passed the ball to him and managed to block out the towering Harris for a moment. The youngster bent his knees and lofted a wild, arching shot that descended through the center of the netless iron hoop. "Oh, yeah. Great job," Shamrock shouted. "Great job." Shamrock wrapped a bear hug around the lad, his eyes lit with joy.

Shamrock tries to make a difference through such personal appearances, through the thousands in donations his family makes to worthy groups, and through his volunteer work in the Lodi area, where he serves as an assistant football coach for the Lodi High School freshman team. He also helps his Dad run the group home for boys in Lockeford, counseling troubled young men, telling them their lives can change for the better, just as his did.

The early evening in Detroit is turning gray and drizzly. The Lincoln glides past Joe Louis Arena, where the marquee announces that the Red Wings are engaged in the hockey play-offs. Producers of the UFC are lucky they set the event for Friday night; there will be no hockey conflict. The next Red Wings game, against Colorado, is set for Sunday. Bob Shamrock maneuvers the car past the Joe Louis memorial, a huge, dangling black fist. The stark monument seems to kindle Ken Shamrock's thoughts about fighting, and about legacy. "I fight because I love it, because I love the competition, the challenge of it," he says. "Fighting is what I do best. I want to be remembered as an all-around champion. I want to be remembered as someone who used technique. Not just power, not just muscle."

Though he is still nursing a broken nose, Shamrock believes he has made good progress in the last two weeks. He is at the weight, 220, that he feels is right. His strength and conditioning have steadily improved. "And my timing is back," he says, punching toward the Lincoln's dashboard, his hands moving in a blur. "My timing is good now." Shamrock does not believe Severn is a particularly adaptive or creative adversary. "He's more defensive. He doesn't try things," says Shamrock. "But this fight will be tougher than the last fight. It's always harder to beat a guy the second time. If they are smart, they've studied you, studied what you do. They are better prepared."

As with nearly every UFC, however, there is some question whether this one will actually take place. County and state prosecutors are trying to stop the fight under an 1869 state law that forbids unlicensed prize fights—a legal artifact held over from the last major era of bare-knuckle fighting. Meyrowritz and his battalion of lawyers have enjoyed uncanny success in meeting and repelling legal opposition to the UFC since the event was created more than two years earlier. Still, Shamrock is unsettled by the continuing legal threats, as groundless as he believes they are. He knows they can result in very personal, very real consequences. Just three weeks earlier, five men who fought in a reality event known as Extreme Fighting, along with the matchmaker, the ring announcer, and the referee, were arrested and jailed following a fight near Montreal. The charge: participating in an illegal bare-knuckle prizefight. The so-called "Extreme Eight" were locked up over the weekend and appeared for an arraignment in handcuffs. As dozens of supporters cheered, the men were released on $1,000 bail each and a promise never to fight or promote such an event in Quebec again.

Somewhere, the ghost of John L. Sullivan is stirring.

Shamrock knows what it is like to be confined to a locked cell. Now, as a father and husband and role model, he has no desire to repeat the experience.

With the Lincoln turned over to parking attendants, the Shamrocks enter the lobby of their hotel, the Westin at the Renaissance Center, and discover several more members of the Shamrock entourage have arrived, the young fighters Jerry Bohlander and Vernon White and Pete Williams. Shamrock will spend more than $10,000 of his own money to fly his fighters and sparring partners to Detroit, to provide them food and hotel rooms. He spent similar amounts in San Juan, in Buffalo, in Casper. It is an investment, he believes, in the education and development of the Lion's Den, whose members he regards as a second family. The only Lion's Den fighter not yet in Detroit is Frank Shamrock, Bob Shamrock's other adoptive son. A rising star on the Pancrase circuit, Frank Shamrock is fighting the rugged Dutchman Bas Rutten in Tokyo. Still, he is scheduled to be in Detroit in time for the fight Friday night.

The young men in the hotel lobby with the Lion's Den logos on their shirts are hungry, eager to venture out for some dinner. "You guys be careful. And don't stay out too late," Shamrock warns the fighters. "The cops are on the look-out for us. They'll arrest you for spitting on the sidewalk."

The Shamrocks have more to do tonight. After an hour to relax and change, Ken and Tina and Bob are interviewed in one of the Westin suites for a CNN program that examines living on the edge. The CNN producer, Peggy Knapp, is a genial but probing interviewer. A parent herself, Knapp is interested in how Shamrock balances being a father and the star of a controversial fighting event.

"I am not ashamed of what I do. I'm proud of what I do," Shamrock says. " And I am proud that my kids know what I do. . . . I love a challenge, I love striving to be the best. Telling kids about fighting is like telling your kids about sex or anything else. You need to educate them. Put things in perspective. Talk about what's right and what's not right."

"The kids know that wrestling is something they do in a dojo," adds Tina. "They do not wrestle in the playground. They do not provoke fights."

Knapp asks the trio about legal efforts to dissolve the UFC. "We are not saying the UFC is for everyone. Ping-pong is not for everyone," Bob says. "But this is America. There is freedom of choice. If you don't want to play ping-pong and you want to play something else, you should be allowed to do that."

The interview lasts nearly an hour. Afterward, Ken and Tina order a light room service dinner. At 9:30, Ken meets some of his fighters in a hotel conference room where wrestling mats have been laid out on the plush carpet. He stretches and then goes through some sparring. "I feel good," he pronounces at the end of the session. "I feel ready." Then he returns to his suite, watches television for a time with Tina, and enjoys a night of dreamless sleep.

Bob, though, will not sleep for a few more hours. When he was a freshman in high school, he resolved to change, to adapt, to reach his fullest potential as a man. Bob Shamrock is still adapting, still reinventing himself. He continues to operate a successful group home for boys, but he has also taken on the daunting responsibility of managing his son's career, and managing, too, the growing business that is Lion's Den.

As his son's manager, he deftly handles numerous chores, from setting up press interviews to negotiating contracts. Shamrock takes care of the many mundane but necessary tasks that arise in the days before a fight. Soon after he arrived in Detroit, for instance, Ken informed his father he was out of the nutritional supplement he favors, a brand carried at General Nutrition Centers. Bob discovered the closest General Nutrition Center was in Ann Arbor. So he drove to the outlying city, purchased the supplement, and drove back, devoting more than two hours to the errand.

Though he was not a fighter himself, Bob Shamrock has keen natural instincts about talent, about a fighter's strengths and weaknesses. He is his son's most candid critic—as well as his most passionate supporter. Though a glib and likable man, he is, like his son, an intense competitor. And he is anything but amiable as he kneels next to the octagon while his son is locked in battle. "When Ken fights, it is time to take care of business," he says. "It is time to do what needs to be done."

Tonight, the night before the fight, Bob Shamrock makes sure everything is in order. Again and again, he reviews the schedule for fight day. He makes certain all members of the entourage have their UFC tickets or passes. He checks to make sure the Pancrase and Lion's Den banners are pressed and ready. And he makes sure, too, that the UFC Superfight belt is polished and bright.

On the morning of Friday, May 17, the day of the Superfight, Ken Shamrock rises at 10:00 A.M. The skies are bleak, promising not a sliver of sunshine. Far below the Shamrock's suite, the Detroit River flows wide and slow and cold, a steady wind chipping at its gray expanse.

As Shamrock awakens and yawns, his wife has a question. "Well, Ken, is it a good day for some butt-kicking?" Shamrock just laughs. He is loose and confident. He feels he is quicker, more skilled and just as strong as his opponent.

Soon, room service waiters roll in a silver cart holding a breakfast of pancakes and eggs and steak, juice and milk. Shamrock eats heavily on the morning of the fight, believing his body needs plenty of fuel for the warfare to come. He will devour more food later, pasta and chicken and salad and bread. He will avoid sugar, convinced it provides only a short and deceptive burst of energy.

Late in the morning, Bob Shamrock enters the suite. He has bad news. Frank has lost in Japan. His fight with Rutten was a ferocious exchange, with Frank at one point driving Rutten through the ropes and out of the ring. But Rutten, a powerful striker and kicker, managed to raise a nasty welt above Shamrock's eye. The ringside doctor halted the fight, so Rutten was declared the victor by a technical knock-out. Frank Shamrock, the provisional King of Pancrase, surrendered his belt to the Dutchman.

In the afternoon, the Shamrocks do a walk-through of Cobo, touring the dungeon-like space that will be Shamrock's dressing room, examining the octagon, doing a quick interview with one of the UFC producers. Then they return to the Westin, to relax and wait. For Ken Shamrock, all is going according to plan. They will return to Cobo at 8:00 P.M., an hour before the first fight, providing plenty of time for Shamrock to dress, stretch, receive a rub-down. There will be no tournament tonight. The format is similar to a boxing card, with six bouts, the final match being the Superfight.

• • •

"You guys are just trying to cover your own butts!" Ken Shamrock should be in a van now, heading to Cobo. Instead, he remains in his hotel suite, sixty-five floors above the Detroit River. He is angry and confused, his body tense as he sits on a cream-colored sofa. Also in the suite are Robert Meyrowitz, Art Davie, Tina Shamrock, and Bob Shamrock.

It is not a happy gathering.

Meyrowitz and Davie are the bearers of grim news. Again, the UFC's lawyers have managed to salvage the event. It will go on, at the time and place scheduled. But just two hours before, Wayne County Circuit Judge Arthur Lombard imposed two rules: no headbutting and no striking with closed fists. Those who step into the octagon and ignore the rules will be subject to arrest, the judge ordered. Meyrowitz has told Shamrock, as he has told the other fighters, that referee John McCarthy will issue warnings. If fighters insist on using fists or head-butts after those repeated warnings, there will be a $50 fine. The fine will be collected at some unspecified point in the future.

Meyrowitz and Davie explain the situation to Shamrock, explain the compromise, explain the way SEG officials intend to react to violations of the judicial order.

"That's just crap," Shamrock says. He believes SEG should not simply threaten fines; he thinks McCarthy should halt a match and disqualify a fighter if he headbutts or strikes with a fist. Shamrock is convinced that SEG is tacitly condoning violation of the law.

Shamrock is in turmoil. He cannot, absolutely will not, violate a judge's order. But he must win the fight. What if Severn violates the order, gains an advantage? What if, as with the fighters in Montreal, he is arrested, led away from the octagon in handcuffs before an audience of four million, including his own children?

"I broke the rules once and I paid the price for it. I tell kids over and over again not to break the rules, not to make the mistakes I made," he tells Meyrowitz. "I am not going to fight under these conditions."

The UFC is set to start in less than forty minutes. Meyrowitz, a businessman trying valiantly to hold his event together, realizes he has said all he can say.

"I have to leave," he tells Shamrock. "The decision is yours."

Shortly after, Shamrock and his entourage depart for Cobo, as well, though no final decision has been made. Shamrock rides to the arena in bitter silence. His Lion's Den fighters know he is upset, though they do not know why. After they have entered the privacy of the dressing room, and the door is tightly shut, Bob Shamrock tells them. They are gathered now, ten men, the Lion's Den fighters, in a tight circle.

"Ken is facing a moral dilemma," Bob Shamrock says. "A judge says there can be no closed-fist strikes, no headbutts. But SEG says the fighters who do that will only be warned and maybe fined."

Above the dressing room, in the arena, the largest crowd ever assembled for a UFC has started to stomp. "WE WANT THE BEAST!

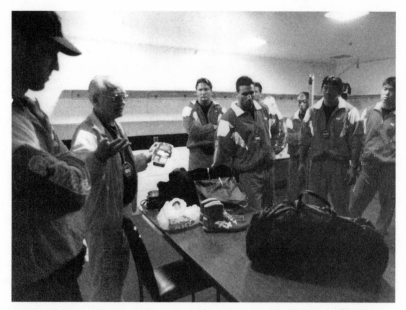

Before the Superfight at Cobo Arena, Bob Shamrock explained to the assembled Lions Den fighters why his son was in anguish over whether or not to fight. *(Calixtro Romias photo)*

WE WANT THE BEAST! WE WANT THE BEAST!"

Shamrock steps forward, into the group of young men. "I don't want to fight for a company that feels it is okay to violate the law," he says. "It's my ass that's on the line. It's my ass that might be thrown into jail." He steps to a training table, where the Superfight belt sits. "I won that belt legally. I won it by fighting within the rules. I will not break the rules to keep it."

Bob Shamrock is in anguish. He understands his son's determination to do what is fair, what is right. But he knows the pressures Meyrowitz and Davie are under. He knows the logic of a compromise that will allow the event to proceed without undue disruptions. "It is my feeling that Ken can fight by the rules and still win. And as far as SEG—no organization is perfect. What do you guys say?," Bob asks.

The elder Shamrock turns first to a Pancrase fighter based in Boston who, among the fighters in the room, has trained with and fought for the Lion's Den the longest. He is a well-spoken man who readily shares his opinion. "Ken, it seems that the judge has put down rules similar to what we do in Pancrase. I think you will win, and that your victory will be even more impressive because you will stick to the rules."

The other men, too, voice their support, their belief that Shamrock can fight and win, win with honor.

Shamrock, though, is not convinced. In his heart, he feels the right thing to do is to leave this arena, leave Detroit, return to his sons, tell them Daddy did not go into the octagon because it was not right. Yet he is here, in the belly of an arena swarming with fans, with television cameras at the ready, with his career and future in the balance.
There seems little choice.

"Okay," he says. "Let's get ready for the fight."

The event begins at 8:00 P.M. As the fights progress, it is clear the participants are paying little attention to the court-imposed rules. Among those watching the fights live in Cobo is Isiah McKinnon, Detroit's chief of police. McKinnon tells a reporter what is obvious: there appear to be violations of the judge's order in these fights, with numerous headbutts and closed-fist strikes. McKinnon, though, will not climb into the octagon and arrest fighters and risk the wrath of thousands. He will make decisions later, he says, after viewing the videotape of the fight.

Halfway across the country, in Lockeford, three boys sit on a living room floor, watched over by their grandparents, Robert and Yolanda Ramirez. The Shamrock boys, Ryan, Connor and Sean, are ready to see their Dad earn his living. But the UFC commentators have not mentioned the judge's order. The boys and their grandparents have no hint of the stress Ken Shamrock is under now.

Shamrock moves to the octagon and reveals not a trace of the pressure, the strain. He appears stoic, invincible. But when the Superfight begins, it does not go according to plan.

Dan Severn, the big wrestler, wearing martial arts gloves, does not charge toward Shamrock, does not even approach him. Instead, he circles, keeps a safe distance, draws Shamrock into a footrace around and around and around the interior of the octagon. Understandably, the fans jeer.

"BOR-RING!," is the chanted assessment of several thousand. No one, even the UFC commentators, can disagree.

"These are two of the best fighters in the world, but they are not fighting," says Don "The Dragon" Wilson, one of the commentators.

"RED WINGS!," begins another chant.

But after Severn tries to lunge at one of his legs, Shamrock drops on the huge man, scrambles for the mounted position, and achieves it. Now he holds the position for more than four minutes, four long minutes when he could land dozens of bloodying, decisive blows. Instead, Shamrock obeys the rules.

Then, leaning back, looking for a submission hold, Shamrock is dislodged by the powerful Severn, who quickly reverses positions. Severn, above Shamrock now, bangs him with his head, then lands glancing blows to Shamrock's face, evoking a trickle of blood.

Drawn by the closed, black-gloved fists, the trickle may prove decisive.

Cobo is roaring now, roaring for The Beast to finish it. But Shamrock holds on, curled up below Severn, avoiding any direct hits.

After twenty-four minutes, the regulation period is over. The fighters rise and return to their handlers. Bob Shamrock knows the fight is close, and he knows that means trouble. No matter that Severn, for most of the fight, had been a jogger, not a warrior. No matter that his son is the champion, and that a challenger, according to the time-honored adage, is supposed to clearly beat a champion to wrest away his belt. With his son's blood on the floor of the octagon and 10,000 fans bellowing for Severn, the judges will not be kind tonight, Bob Shamrock knows. "You are losing," he shouts to his son. "You are letting him win. You have to go after him."

During two overtime periods, as a hamburger and four beer cups descend into the octagon, Shamrock chases again. Severn runs again. With a few seconds remaining, Shamrock shoots in and tries for a leg submission. It is too late. ·

The Superfight is over.

On a vote of two to one, the judges agree, as Bob Shamrock suspected they would, to give Dan Severn the shiny brass belt.

In the locker room, the Lion's Den fighters gather again around Shamrock, their friend, their coach, their brother. Shamrock is soaked with sweat. His hair is a slickened tangle. There is redness over his left eye. Some of the fighters are screaming their disgust at the decision, a decision they believe rewarded a man for avoiding a fight, not winning one.

But time and time again, Shamrock has told his fighters to win and lose with grace. It is time to underline the lesson.

"Hold on. Hold on," he says, looking into the faces of the fighters. "The decision tonight was the right decision. Dan Severn fought a smart fight. I expected him to come after me. He didn't. But I did not go after him, either. I accept the decision. There will be another day." The fighters are quiet for a moment. Then, one-by-one, his Lion's Den brothers break into applause for Ken Shamrock. The applause builds until the cluttered cubicle resounds.

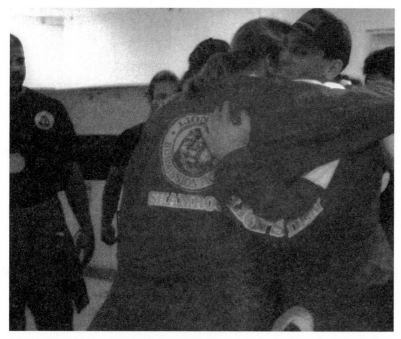

Shamrock did not win the Superfight with Dan Severn, but he retained the admiration and respect of his Lions Den fighters. (Calixtro Romias photo)

Shamrock embraces his wife, his Dad, and each of his fighters. As he wraps his arms around Bohlander, the young fighter tells Shamrock, "It takes more to make a champion than a belt." Then Shamrock showers and rides in the shuttle van back to the Westin Hotel, where he and his wife ascend to the sixty-fifth floor. As soon as he enters the suite, Shamrock walks to the phone and calls Lockeford, California, to speak with three little boys. He tells each one he loves them, that he and their mommy and Grandpa and Uncle Frank are coming home the next day. As the end of the conversation, Ryan, at eight years old the oldest, and well-versed on ways of the UFC, asks a question. "Daddy, you could have hit him. But you didn't hit him. Why didn't you hit him Daddy?," Ryan asks. Shamrock smiles. "I chose not to, Ryan," he says. "I chose not to hit him. It's a little complicated. But I will explain it all when we get home." He wishes his son sweet dreams and hangs up the phone.

Kenneth Wayne Shamrock, child of rage, has prevailed.

PART TWO

Inside the Lion's Den

The Secrets of Submission Fighting

by Ken Shamrock

Chapter 16

Do or Die
Welcome to the Lion's Den

"What makes Lion's Den so successful is not just Ken Shamrock's determination to win, but his determination to learn."

—Maurice Smith, Extreme Fighting heavyweight champion
and world heavyweight kickboxing champion

Welcome to Lion's Den. Now get ready to fight. I don't mean doing kata until you're bored out of your mind. And I don't mean breaking boards or sparring with heavy pads on.

I mean fighting—as in combat, hand-to-hand, no holds barred. The blood may flow and the bones may break. Sound savage? Well, it's what the martial arts were all about in the beginning: fighting to win, fighting to protect your honor, and maybe your land or even your family. This is what you might face in a bar or on the street when some drunk takes a swing at you. It's what I've faced in Pancrase Hybrid Wrestling matches in Japan, where some of the best martial artists on the planet converge to rock and rumble. And it's the type of warfare you can find in the Ultimate Fighting Championship (UFC), the mixed martial arts event where I claimed the Superfight Championship in 1995.

At the dojo I founded, Lion's Den, we've developed fighters who have dominated the world of no-holds-barred competition. We have fought and won in Pancrase, the UFC, the Hawaiian Superbrawl, and the Michigan Clash of the Dragons. No dojo is as successful, and no dojo is as intense.

Though I have recently returned to pro-wrestling, Lion's Den reflects my background in full-contact fighting. I've fought and won in alleys and bars. I've hit guys on the football field, in basic training for the U.S. Marines, and in toughman contests. I've refined my skills in Pancrase matches and the UFC. I have God-given strength and quickness. And I have an anger that still smolders deep inside, an anger

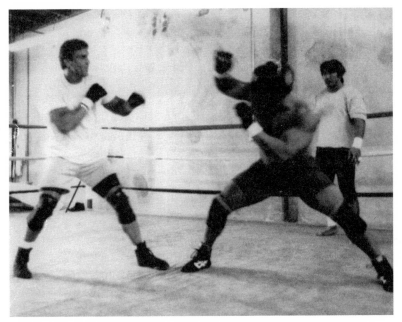

We do not do kata in the Lion's Den. We do not bow to one another. We fight. *(Calixtro Romias photo)*

that for a long time never let me back down or give up. But I'm not a great fighter because of these things. I am a great fighter because I have never stopped listening or learning.

To become a master, you must always be a student. Always. From every fight, whether it was my first Toughman contest in a dusty rodeo arena or my UFC Superfight against Royce Gracie, I have walked away with something new, something about myself, about fighting, or both. I have learned from every victory and from every loss. Let me say this right here and right now: you don't become great without losing—John L. Sullivan lost, Ali wasn't unbeaten, neither was Joe Louis, and neither am I. In the world of martial arts, if somebody tells you they are undefeated, it probably means one of two things. Either they are a liar, or they haven't been in enough tough fights.

I have been in a lot of fights, more than I can remember. I have fought in group homes where I was raised as a kid, in high school where I learned to wrestle, in bars where I worked as a bouncer, in back alleys where I fought bare-knuckle for a wad of cash slapped on the hood of a pick-up. I learned a lot on the street, but I learned a lot more when I went to Japan and started fighting in Pancrase matches. I learned how to eat right and train right. And I learned a system based on submission techniques, which I believe is the most effective fighting system around. I've reshaped the system and built on it. And I've showcased it in my matches in the UFC.

It is this system, the way of fighting, training, and developing mental toughness, that I share with the young studs I work with at the Lion's Den, in Lodi, California.

We don't train at the Lion's Den for trophies, colored belts, or stress relief. We train to win the toughest hand-to-hand combat sport events in the world. Inside the Lion's Den we have tested one another and bloodied one another. We have broken each other's bones, and torn our tendons. We have toughened one another for battle. And like soldiers who have gone through war together, we have a bond, a kinship. Lion's Den is more than a dojo: it is a state of mind, a family of fighters. And we are, in my humble opinion, the best in the world.

So, if you want to learn about the essence of martial arts, step into the Lion's Den. If you want to strengthen whatever fighting system you now use, step into the Lion's Den. And if you want to be ready if some beered-up yahoo takes a swing at you in the parking lot of a convenience store, step into the Lion's Den.

I will teach you, train you, and I will make you as ready as you can be. My tone at times may seem harsh, even cocky. However, I have the greatest respect for my fighters as well as those from other dojos. As a personal principle, I do not put people down. I strongly believe in treating people the way you yourself want to be treated. But I am direct. I can be blunt. I am demanding. You will appreciate this the next time you do battle, either in a dojo, in a ring, or on the street.

First, a warning. I tell everyone who enters our dojo this: I don't give a shake if you are weak or clumsy or slow. But I demand that you give me your best. I demand that you show me heart. When I tell you to do something, don't say you will try. In the Lion's Den, it's do or die.

Welcome to the Lion's Den. Consider yourself part of the family.

Chapter 17

Food for Battle
Building the Body of a Warrior

"We eat and work out. Then we eat. Then we work out. Then we eat some more."

—Frank Shamrock, top-ranked Pancrase fighter
and overseer of the Lion's Den fighters' home.

To create the body of a warrior, you need good materials in the right portions. I will now talk about what you should feed your body. I don't want to sound self-righteous. I do take my wife, Tina, and my kids to Taco Bell from time to time like anyone else. We enjoy an occasional pizza. And I have a weakness for Carl's Jr. Western BBQ burgers. More often than not, however, I watch what I eat very carefully. If I splurge, I am very aware of it.

I demand that my fighters follow a strict eating regimen. You don't build or maintain a fighter's body on fudge and potato chips. You build it with a well-balanced diet that includes plenty of protein and carbohydrates and a lesser portion of sugar and fat.

If you step into the fighters' house where Lion's Den recruits live, you will probably find them eating. They eat solid meals four or five times a day, plus snacks, and drink a lot of juice and water. They do not get fat. While they may gain weight, it is muscle and not slop. At the rate they build muscle and burn fuel, my problem is usually keeping them from dropping weight. I keep the house stocked with good food, quality food, and plenty of it.

All of us drink nutritional shakes, one or two a day. These drinks help build muscle and keep your weight up. There are a lot of brands out there. I don't want to single one out. Find one you like, one that works for you, and stick with it. We also drink water, and lots of it. Most of us carry a bottle of water around and sip on it throughout the day. With all the training and sparring we do, we lose an ocean of sweat. We have to stay hydrated.

You will always find fresh fruit in the fighter's house, including

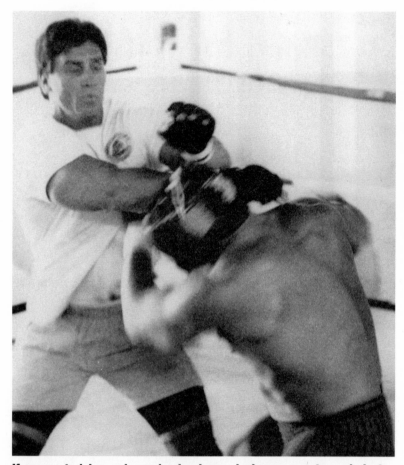

If you are training and sparring hard, your body craves water and plenty of calories, most of them from carbohydrates and protein, some from fat, few from sugar. Here I'm sparring with Mike Radnov, a former wrestler who helped me prepare for my second Superfight with Dan Severn. (Calixtro Romias photo)

apples, bananas, and oranges. You will find gallons of fruit juice, mountains of rice, and enough chicken breasts to feed an army. Chicken and rice, with some vegetables and seasoned with soy sauce, is probably the most common meal served in the house. Chicken is consumed for protein, to build and maintain the muscle for striking, kicking, and submission fighting. Rice is consumed for the complex carbohydrates that fuel the battle. Vegetables are consumed for the vitamins, minerals, and fiber.

Most of the fighters eat a large breakfast which includes oatmeal or pancakes, juice, toast, eggs—a blend of protein and carbohydrates.

They do not drink coffee since it acts as a diuretic and dries you up. After a workout, they come back to the house and eat again, this time a meal heavy in protein, including chicken, milk, fruit, more eggs, maybe a peanut butter sandwich. A couple of hours later, they will usually snack on apples or bananas and have a protein shake. Before the night workout session they will eat again. As with the others, this meal will be a blend of protein and carbohydrates, including pasta, maybe fish, a big salad, some fruit, and cottage cheese. After their second workout, they come back and devour even more chicken or fish with rice, broccoli, carrots, and juice. Some of the guys like their baked or mashed potatoes instead of rice, which is fine.

That is pretty much the regimen we follow. We take in a steady stream of water, consume tons of chicken, fish, eggs, fruits, veggies, turkey and tuna sandwiches, pasta, oatmeal, and toast. Again, we stress balance and variety. Steak, turkey, halibut, or shrimp sometimes substitutes for chicken breast. Baked potatoes or even French fries may be slipped in instead of rice.

Be sure not to scoop in the fat, but don't try to train without it, either. You need some fat to maintain your energy and strength and keep your joints loose. If you get too lean and hard, your joints can actually start aching. Your tendons will also become tighter and easier to tear or snap. So, a peanut butter sandwich or some fries aren't poison—they just need to be a part of the overall diet, not the main portion.

The Lion's Den regimen changes on Fridays, when the fighters get to eat what they want: burgers, doughnuts, pie, burritos, whatever. Most of the guys appreciate the chance to indulge a little, and few of them do it to excess. If you are working out hard and often, and your diet is fundamentally good, you can splurge and get away with it. Just be aware of what you are eating and how much. Keep it in balance.

You can almost always find me with a water bottle. It's very important to stay hydrated, especially before and after training and before fights. Here I'm taking a break in a training dojo before my Superfight with Kimo Leopoldo in Puerto Rico. (Lions Den photo)

We don't keep alcohol in the fighters' house, but we aren't teeto-
talers, either. The guys can have a beer or a glass of wine on Friday
nights, or if they are out socially. Again, they do not consume to
excess.

On the day of a fight, I eat more than usual, including an especially large breakfast. Your body needs plenty of ammunition for the
war ahead. If I am fighting at 8:00 p.m., for example, I usually get up
around 10:00 a.m. and have eggs, toast, potatoes, fruit, and juice.
Sometimes I'll have a steak with my eggs. You want to be loading carbohydrates into your body throughout the day. I will have a sandwich
and fruit and maybe a salad around noon. I eat again in the late afternoon, around three or four o'clock, maybe pasta or rice and chicken
with bread and vegetables. A couple of hours before the fight, I'll
have an apple and banana—they are light and digestible and add
more complex carbohydrates. This all may sound like a lot, but if you
have been in serious and demanding training, your body will be soak-
ing in the carbohydrates and nutrients as fast as you can pour them
in. You must also be sure to give your body enough fuel to make it
through a long battle that will steadily draw on your storehouse of
energy. On fight day especially, watch the sweets. They are empty
calories. They will cause you to flare up quick, expend too much
energy, and burn out.

On the day of a fight you want to drink water, and lots and lots of
it. If you are fighting in the heat, as I did in Puerto Rico against Kimo
Leopoldo, you need to drink even larger quantities. You also need to
drink more if you are fighting at a high altitude or if you've traveled
by jet in the last day or two. Elevation and jet travel both tend to
dehydrate the body.

After a fight, grab that water bottle again, but don't gulp a huge
shot at once. Drink some, drink a little more, and eventually just start
sipping again. Give your body the chance to make use of the moisture
that's seeping into you.

To recap: eat a good balanced diet tilted toward protein and carbohydrates, with a moderate amount of fat and a minimal amount of
sugar. Don't fret too much about splurging now and then, as long as
you are training hard and your diet is on track you will be okay. If you
are in heavy training, consider nutritional supplement drinks. Always
be sure to sip a steady supply of water.

I have been asked many times how anabolic steroids might fit
into a fighter's overall plan of diet and training. The answer is simple:
they don't. Steroids have a place in legitimate medical and veterinary

settings. Many don't know this, but when I was first active in pro-wrestling years ago, I had some experience with steroids. Steroids can rapidly enlarge muscle mass. Muscle mass, in exertion, rapidly burns up huge amounts of oxygen and fuel. A no-holds-barred fighter who's ballooned up with steroids can't last longer than a few minutes. No real fighter swollen-up with steroids will win, at least not regularly. I do not use steroids anymore. I don't allow my fighters to use them. either. Steroids are not welcome in the Lion's Den. Period.

Chapter 18

Combat Tough
Getting Strong, Flexible, and Callused

"Ken Shamrock . . . has the strength of a non-mortal."
—*Black Belt,* July 1996

My Ultimate Fighting Championship Superfight against Royce Gracie turned into a siege. Gracie is a lean Brazilian ju-jitsu fighter who doesn't carry much extra bulk. We struggled for more than thirty-six minutes. At the end Royce was battered and beat down; I wasn't even breathing hard.

In my Superfight against Kimo Leopoldo, a 270-pound brawler from Hawaii, I used power and agility to lock him in a knee bar and cause him to tap out. I forced Patrick Smith, another big, tough fighter, to tap out with an ankle hook. And I forced Dan "The Beast" Severn, a massive Greco-Roman wrestler, to tap out with a guillotine choke. Those fights all ended in less than five minutes. In addition, I have been in Toughman contests and street fights that lasted less than 30 seconds.

Whether it's a fight in a saloon or a championship event in an octagon in front of six million people, you have to be ready for anything. With timing and strength alone you may be able to knock out or choke out your opponent in seconds. But you may have to dig in for a battle against a defender like Gracie or Oleg Taktarov and prevail through guts and conditioning.

Some of the submissions techniques I will discuss here can by used by anybody, anywhere. Somebody who is jumped in a parking lot or in a bar can make use of submissions basics without full-scale training. But as we use it in professional fighting, submissions demands unusual strength and stamina. This is another way the Lion's Den differs from other dojos. We don't hold aerobics classes and we aren't into kata. We are preparing for no-holds-barred battles the world over. Every part of a submissions fighter's body has to be in tune. He needs superb upper body strength for striking and grappling. Submissions fighters need extra power because they often go for control and submissions holds on

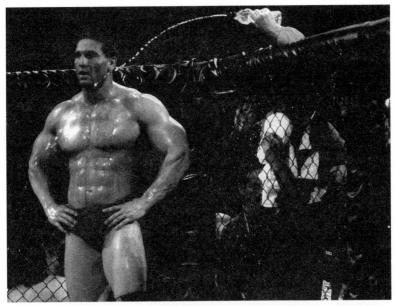

You need a strong upper body to fight in the octagon. But as a submission fighter, your legs need to be powerful, too. Here my dad tries to cool me off during a break in a Superfight. *(Calixtro Romias photo)*

an opponent's legs, which are bigger, stronger, and more difficult to control than arms. You have to be able to grip, lock, and load a sizable limb whose owner is not always eager to go along with the program.

While this takes muscle strength, you also need stamina. In a tournament, you might have to fight two or three guys to make the finals. It's grueling. Sometimes you can't predict whether you are going to fight for three minutes or thirty, and you don't want to battle your way through the preliminaries only to be wasted for the big finale. You have to be ready, ready for anything. At the Lion's Den, we always train for the toughest possible scenario, and then we push beyond.

So, before you learn submissions techniques you need to toughen your body. In the first few weeks of our program, the "young boys" can barely walk because their legs are so sore. Their stomachs hurt, their arms and shoulders are aching all of the time. The little plastic buckets are always ready for anybody who starts to puke. Their muscles are waking up with a scream. Even muscles they never knew existed are coming alive. But the pain slowly goes away, and their bodies become muscular and hard. This is part of the process we call callusing. This means making parts of your body tough and resistant to pain and injury. For instance, before one of our fighters is callused, his mouth will hurt a lot and sometimes bleed. Once he's callused, after his mouth has been exposed to the grinding work of submissions sparring, the pain goes away and he will seldom bleed. In essence, fighters must callous everything, including muscles, tendons, and ligaments. Especially in submission fighting, the soft and connective tissue needs to be not only elastic, but tough like rawhide.

Mental callousing is an important part of becoming a better fighter, too. If you are mentally calloused, you won't panic when you feel your leg being twisted. You don't freak out when somebody is trying to sink in a choke around your neck. You know how far your body can go, how much you can take before you must physically give up. That threshold is much further than most beginning fighters think it is.

But back to conditioning. After three months, our guys can do 500 squats, 100 push-ups and 100 stomach crunches consecutively. They can fight for an hour or more without a break. They are among the strongest and best-conditioned fighters anywhere. I would wager that there are very few professional athletes in the world who are in Lion's Den kind of shape. And while we do use weights and weight machines, and we have the benefit of a dojo, most of our work can be done in a garage or even a living room.

A submissions fighter, or anyone fighting full-contact, must keep this in mind: you are only as strong as your weakest part. You must bring your entire body (calves, quadriceps, abdominal, chest, biceps, triceps, neck, and back) up to the highest possible level of fitness. The parts must all work together. In a sense, your body is a machine. A weak part can break down and damage everything. You do not want to blow out a piston in the middle of a fight.

I tell my fighters that ninety-percent of a fight is the preparation. If you enter a fight physically and mentally ready, you will usually win. If you don't, well, good luck. I can't stress this point too much. If you are a competitive fighter, you must struggle to get your body and mind ready for the fight, which takes time and discipline. Through conditioning, you will gain confidence about your ability to control an opponent, to absorb punishment, to persevere through a tough fight. There is a lot said these days about self-esteem. When your body is hard and flexible, your sense of self-esteem for fighting will greatly improve.

You don't need any fancy equipment to start your conditioning. A light, loose T-shirt, a pair of gym shorts, and a pair of good-quality cross-training shoes will do fine. We don't wear gis in the Lion's Den, though we sometimes train with them to prepare for a certain opponent. In my view, gis, especially in a long fight, make a fighter heavier, slower, and hotter. Yes, they have advantages and can be used effectively to help choke an opponent. In addition, because they are heavy canvas, they can also be used to slice or chafe an opponent. However, they can also be used against you, so we don't bother wearing them.

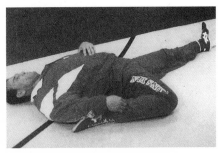

Figure 1

Always begin your workout by stretching and warming up for at least fifteen minutes. Always. If you don't, you may seriously injure your muscles or tendons. Use the warm-up time to think about the workout, sparring, or the fight to follow. When you warm up, begin to consciously regulate your breathing. By controlling your breath, you can force yourself to relax and conserve your mental and physical energy. Get in the habit of being aware of your breathing patterns. Controlled breathing is key to being loose and patient.

A good way to warm up is to go for a light jog, nothing fast or furious. Just jog for half-a-mile or so, maybe around the block twice, or a short route near your dojo. Jogging will get your heartbeat up, loosen your joints and muscles. There is minimum danger of pulling a muscle while jogging, as opposed to sprinting. Remember to keep it loose and short, just enough to break a light sweat.

We continue the warm-up by dropping to the floor and doing the hurdler's stretch. To do this, tuck one leg under your buttocks and extend the other one in front of you (Fig. 1). From this position, gently reach your hands toward your toes, which will stretch your hamstrings. After a few stretches in this position, switch legs and continue stretching. When you feel fairly loose, lean back until your head is on the mat, which will stretch your quadriceps. The hurdler's stretch is good for loosening your hamstrings, quadriceps, calves, and back.

Another warm-up, and an important one, is the neck bridge (Fig. 2). To do this, lie on your back with the top of your head on the floor. Using your hands for balance, arch your back. Doing this will build the strength and flexibility in your neck necessary for withstanding choke holds.

Pancrase and UFC fans often comment on my well-developed upper body. I do have a strong chest and fair-sized biceps. I can bench press more than 500 pounds, and I can press 250 pounds 50 times without stopping. But my legs are even stronger. In fact, the first thing

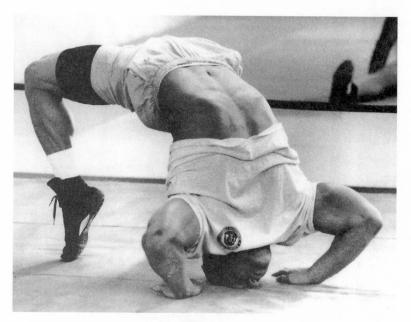

Figure 2

we stress to our young fighters is the importance of lower body strength. Strong legs put more power in your kicks. But even more important, your legs give you the strength to shoot in and take an opponent down. Your legs give you the power on the ground to turn and control an opponent. And your legs give you the stamina to outlast the man you are fighting. In submission fighting, your legs are your foundation. If you don't have a strong foundation, the house is shaky.

After you are warmed up, it is time to begin submissions training. In explaining how to do this, old Sammy Saranaka had it right when he stated that squats are a great way to both test and build your endurance. So, begin your training with at least fifty squats and build, build, build. If you can't do fifty, try this: stand in a doorway and place your hands on the door frame. Then, using your hands to help with balance and to pull you up, do the squats. If you can do more than fifty, great, do more. It is essential to do as many as it takes to get your quadriceps burning and your lungs puffing. If you have to stop frequently, try repeating sets of twenty-five or more until you can do them continuously, without stopping.

Since squats build lower body stamina and strength so well, they may be the single most important way to prepare your body for submission fighting, as well as other martial arts. They are excellent because you can do them rain or shine, night or day. As I have stated earlier, the fighters at Lion's Den can do at least 500 squats in a row. You should spend at least half-an-hour doing squats, especially in the beginning, to build your legs into the strong, supple base you need them to be. Push yourself to your limit. In a fight or in competition, you'll be glad you did.

A variation of the squat is the jump-squat (Figs. 3, 4). In this exercise, drop low, swinging your hands down toward your feet. Then jump up, arching your feet and calves and shooting your hands up. You should be jumping six inches to a foot off the ground with each jump-squat. These are excellent for the explosive movements of submissions fighting. These go quickly. Try doing sets of twenty-five, working up to fifty or more. Have a partner count them out for you. Then take a break and count for him. Working out with a partner makes the drill go faster. It's more fun, too.

A priority for squats and other conditioning exercises is to always be sure to maintain the proper form. If you get loose and sloppy, you will fight loose and sloppy. If you tire and find yourself performing the exercise improperly, take a break until you can continue with the exercise correctly.

Another tried-and-true way to develop lower body strength is running. Now I'm no marathoner, but when I competed in track and field in high school, I did the sprints, the pole vault, and the discus. Just about everything except the distance races—they were too long and too boring for me. However, I do run for distance now, in part because it builds stamina and strength, and because it adds variety to

Figure 3, 4

my workouts. Still, I don't claim to be a Frank Shorter and you don't have to be either. Try running one mile a few times a week. Work up to two miles, and then to three. I try to run three miles three times a week. Sometimes I substitute running the stairs at a local stadium, as it is a great way to shape and define your quadriceps and build your endurance. Vary your running according to your mood. If you feel

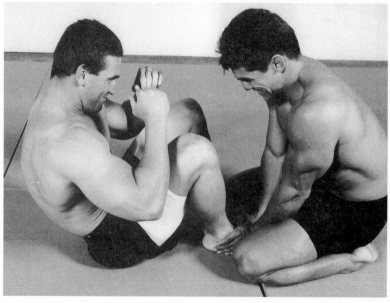

Figure 5

good, gallop at a brisk pace. If not, take it slow and steady. If you are
going to take a long run, start out with a light jog, just as you would
for most of your workouts. Don't forget to work variety into your work-
outs. An example would be to cut your run short and jump rope for
ten or twenty minutes. You will be surprised at how fast jumping rope
can get you winded. Jumping rope increases your stamina and your
timing.

Let's move up the body. Lion's Den fighters are known for their
great abdomens. I have a pretty fair six-pack of abs, and my brother
Frank's are even more heavily chiseled. It is essential to build good
abs, and it seems everybody is buying some contraption to get their
stomach muscles in shape. We don't build a hardened gut for cos-
metics—we do it because a strong abdomen is absolutely critical to
one's ability to fight long and hard.

Think about it: your abs connect the upper and lower body, like
a hinge. If your hinge is weak, it doesn't matter how strong your gate
or fence is, you are not going to swing for too long. Strong abs are
essential for allowing your lower and upper body to work in unison,
an important part of submission fighting. And think about this, too:
your stomach is one of the parts of your body most vulnerable to
attack. You can get hit in the arm, shoulder, even the back of a head,
and not suffer much damage. But, if you take a shot in the gut, you

will most likely feel it. So protect your vulnerable belly by covering it with a hard shield of muscle.

Again, we don't do much that is fancy. We haven't bought or used any of those plastic gadgets you see on television. We do crunches, and

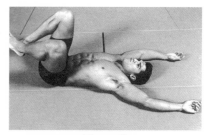

Figure 6

hundreds of them. We do them slowly, exhaling every time, making certain to use the muscles to their maximum potential (Fig. 5). If you do 200 crunches a day, your paunch will quickly melt away and become a washboard of steel. Think of this as your flak jacket. Many parts of our workout, such as squats and even running, indirectly strengthen the abs. But the crunches quickly and steadily build your shield and keep it hard and tough.

You can also try the reverse crunch as a variation (Fig. 6). To do this, lie on your back with your arms stretched up and flat against the floor or mat. Swing your knees up toward your chest. Do a set of ten to start, then move up to five sets of ten.

Now let's move to the upper body. You will need strength here for strikes, grappling, and submission holds. Start with something really fundamental, like push-ups. Yes, we do push-ups at the Lion's Den. We also do chin-ups. Start with whatever number you can do before getting shaky and breaking form. Then, over the next few weeks, steadily build your endurance until you can do at least fifty push-ups and twenty chin-ups without stopping. You will be on your way to Lion's Den-style condition in no time.

You can achieve a good level of strength through these exercises, but our fighters also work out with weights at least three times a week. If you are serious about your fighting shape, I recommend that you too consider pumping iron. Again, it is essential to maintain the proper form at all times when lifting weights. You want to keep a smooth, controlled action throughout each lift. If you start losing muscle control, stop, recover, and then push yourself a little more. You will progress faster if you maintain proper form. You will also develop better overall discipline.

Remember, if you are sharp in your conditioning, you will be sharp in a fight. If you are sloppy in conditioning, your fight will be a mess. Again, I want to stress that the fight is in the preparation.

When our young boys start out, some can barely bench press

150 pounds. In a couple of months, most are up to between 300 and 400 pounds. We try to blend mass weight with repetitions, however. The goal is not to simply lift a mountain of iron, but to get very, very strong while building endurance and maintaining flexibility.

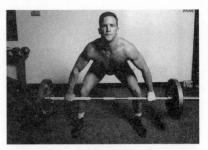

Figure 7

I suggest that when lifting weights you use a progressive system called "pyramiding." To do this, start with a weight that you can comfortably lift five times. Take a short breather and then add five pounds and do four repetitions. Take another short breather, add five more pounds, and do three repetitions. Take another breather, add five more pounds, then do two repetitions. Take another breather, again add an additional five pounds and do one final, mighty lift. You should have to strain to complete the final lift. It should be the most you can heft while maintaining good form. After two weeks of using this progression, try to increase

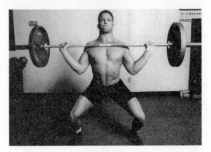

Figure 8

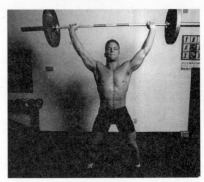

Figure 9

the weight by ten pounds for each set of repetitions. This will give you a good ratio of repetitions to mass weight. Try to lift at least three times a week.

We also do a lot of squats with weights on our shoulders, which greatly builds your leg strength. A great way we build both leg and upper body strength is the clean and press. To perform this exercise, drop down and grip the bar about two to three inches outside your shoulder width. Do not jerk the weight up, but lift gradually with your legs and hips until the weight is tensing your arms and you have to take the slack out of your arms and legs. Now you can quickly heft the

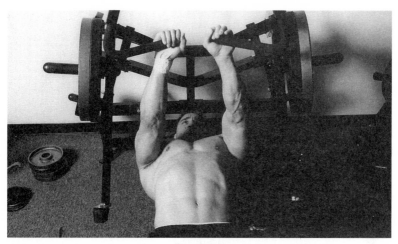

Figure 10

weight up to your shoulder's height (Figs. 7, 8). Next, in an explosive motion, push the barbell high above your head, extending your arms (Fig. 9). Keep your feet a shoulder's width apart and use your legs top drive the weight up. Bring the weight down to the height of your shoulder again, and then bring it back to the floor. To build the chest and arms, we do bench presses and arm curls (Figs. 10–12). Again, use the pyramiding system of adding weight progressively until you cannot maintain form. It's important, especially after you've been lifting for six weeks or so, to work the weights intensively. You don't need countless

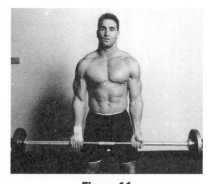

Figure 11

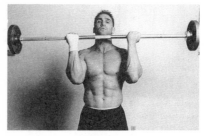

Figure 12

reps to get strong, but you do need to push it, to lift as much as you can lift.

It is a lot of work running, jumping rope, doing squats, push-ups, chin-ups, and lifting weights. However, if you stick with it you will be flexible, strong, and calloused. You will then be prepared to fight.

Chapter 19

Scramble

Drills to Make You Quick and Agile

"Ken is so quick, so explosive. Just when you think you have him, bam! He's going for a choke or a submission hold."

—Dan Freeman, former sparring partner,
AAU Mr. California bodybuilder, and karate black belt.

A
s I fought Kimo Leopoldo in UFC XIII, there were a few moments where neither one of us was in control. At one point, I saw a chance for a leg submission, and I went all-out to achieve it. Kimo knew what I was doing and rolled desperately to keep me from controlling his leg. Both of us were moving very fast, our muscles and minds were in continuous motion.

During a freestyle fight, the time when both competitors are actively trying to outmaneuver one another is called a scramble. You have to be ready to scramble, to use your balance, your flexibility, and your speed to decisively seize an offensive or defensive position. It is

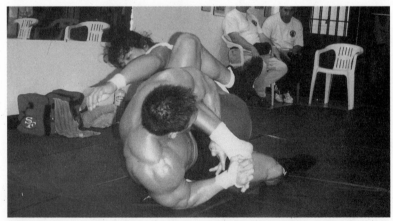

There are times when neither fighter has a clear advantage and both are moving quickly for position. Here I am scrambling for position against Funaki in a grappling session, working to apply a toehold. *(Lions Den photo)*

a little like being in a so-called "dog fight"—you are either rushing to get your opponent into the crosshairs to shoot him out of the sky, or you are moving like crazy to veer out of the line of fire, survive, and mount your own offensive.

At the Lion's Den we have a series of drills and special exercises designed to help us stay limber and flexible. They help us develop a strong sense of balance, and to move explosively and reflexively when we scramble.

We do these movements time and time again, until they become second nature. These drills and exercises all have practical applications. When you practice the duck walk, for example, you are helping prepare for a powerful shoot that will quickly and cleanly topple your opponent. The rope and leap-frog drills help you curl and roll, either to escape a hold or to achieve one of your own. If you practice these movements frequently, they will occur automatically during a fight. Following is a brief description of the drills and special exercises we use at the Lion's Den.

The Rope Drill

The rope drill develops explosiveness, balance, agility, and coordination. While you will start by jumping over the rope, you will end up scooting under it. The drill strengthens your quadriceps, hamstrings, and calves. To begin, face the rope with your feet about a

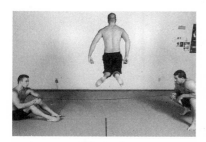

Figure 1

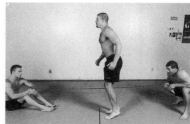

Figure 2

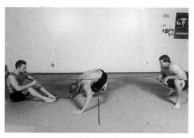

Figure 3

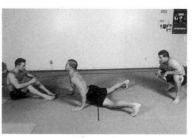

Figure 4

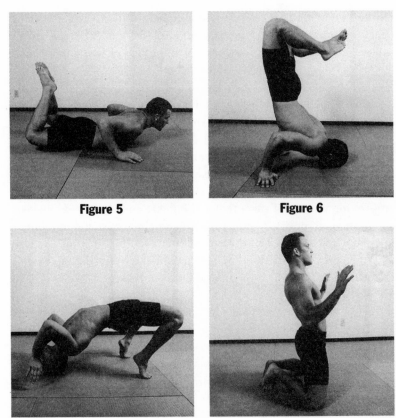

Figure 5

Figure 6

Figure 7

Figure 8

shoulders-width apart. Jump forward over the rope, then jump over the rope backwards (Fig. 1). For maximum results, do not turn around as you leap. For best results, do this ten consecutive times while maintaining good form.

Next, stand sideways to the rope with your feet about a shoulders-width apart. Jump over the rope and back again (Fig. 2) in a single crisp, clean motion. Repeat this ten times also.

Finally, jump over the rope sideways, then lean down, dive under the rope (Fig. 3), and come up on the other side (Fig. 4). As you dive under the rope, spread your legs apart, as if sprawling. Ten repetitions will do it.

For maximum benefit, do all three rope drills in a row as described above, with no rest in between.

Belly Roll to Back Bridge
The belly roll to back bridge will help you build flexibility and

balance. It also strengthens the neck. It is a fairly advanced drill, so do not be frustrated if it takes a few sessions to get the feel for it. Begin by rolling on your belly and then kicking your legs up above your head (Fig. 5). It is important as you roll on your belly to arch your back; this helps build the momentum to get your legs up and moving (Fig. 6). Now flip over so you are bridging your neck (Fig. 7). Finally, shove off with your hands, swing your torso over your feet until you are in a kneeling position (Fig. 8). Do this in a fluid motion, maintaining momentum throughout the drill. Once you get the knack, do this eight to ten times.

Nip-ups

Nip-ups are short, explosive exercises that stress balance. Start by leaning low over the floor (Fig. 9). Tuck your head, put your hands on the floor (Fig. 10), and roll forward. As you roll, kick out with your legs and spring up with your hands (Fig. 11). If you do this right, you will land on your feet in a very crisp, quick motion (Fig. 12). Tuck and

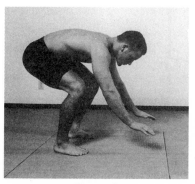

Figure 9

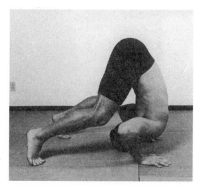

Figure 10

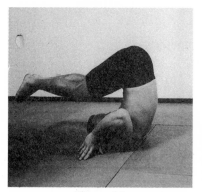

Figure 11

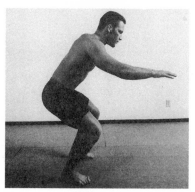

Figure 12

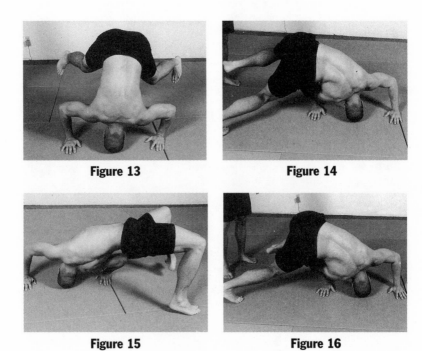

Figure 13   Figure 14

Figure 15   Figure 16

repeat. Do two or three reps across the ring or practice area, then come back to the starting position.

Walk Around Drill

The walk around helps build your neck strength and flexibility. This is important in submissions fighting, as a strong neck will help you slip a choke. It will also help you avoid neck injuries, which I can tell you from personal experience are not uncommon in grappling. The drill also helps build agility as well as balance. In freestyle fighting, balance is everything. You can't kick or strike powerfully without being balanced. In a freestyle scramble, you may be flipped upside down. You may be tucking and rolling several times. Like being in the cockpit of a fighter jet, you need to know where you are at all times. You must be balanced, oriented to your surroundings and your opponent, and preparing for attack.

To do the walk around drill, squat and put you head on the mat, placing your hands on the floor on each side of your head (Fig. 13). Your hands are important, especially when you start out, to keep your balance. Now move your legs so you are "walking" in a clockwise direction. Keep your head in the same position. After several steps, you will have to flip your legs over (Fig. 14). Now continue to walk in a clockwise direction (Figs. 15, 16). Do this once or twice to start. Over time, you can walk up to ten or more full rotations. This is another tough drill, but a critical one. Don't worry if you slip or fall at first. Stick with it, and you will develop a neck like a bull.

The Duck Walk

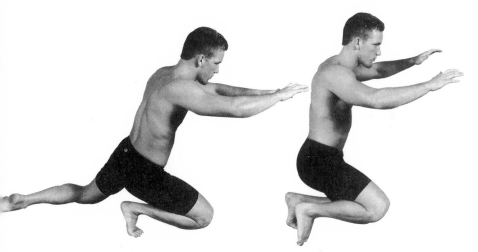

Figure 17   **Figure 18**

Just like it sounds, you walk low, sort of like waddling. The lower, the better, as long as you maintain your balance. To do this, bend your knees (Fig. 17) and stride forward, with your knees barely grazing over the floor (Fig. 18). Keep your arms extended in front of you, shoulder-high, like you do when you shoot in on somebody, and keep your back held as straight as possible. This is demanding on your quads, but greatly helps with developing and maintaining balance. Try duck walking in relatively short, steady sets. We usually duck walk ten times across the mat in our dojo, a distance of about thirty feet. As you duck walk, visualize yourself shooting in on your opponent.

Cartwheels

We do cartwheels, just like kids do. They help develop balance and shoulder and arm strength. They are also helpful in maintaining flexibility, something you need to keep in mind as you build muscle mass. Start by standing with your feet about a shoulder's width apart. Next, lower one hand to the floor (Fig. 19) while flipping your feet up

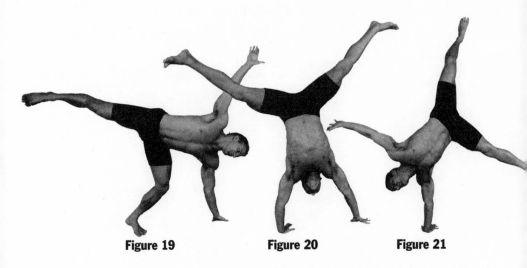

Figure 19   **Figure 20**   **Figure 21**

and over your head. As your momentum carries you forward, place your other hand on the floor (Fig. 20), swing your legs all the way around (Fig. 21) and back to the floor. Kids make these look easy, but they may take some practice. Try to perform a cartwheel that is smooth, with your legs held in control over your head, and a crisp, graceful landing. Do a few cartwheels across your dojo and back again. Three or four sets is fine.

Leap Frog Drill

Another great way to develop balance and control of movement in the leap frog drill. In this two-man exercise, one man squats with his legs apart and his elbows on his knees. The other man places his palms on the man's back and leaps over (Fig. 22). (Make sure your legs are spread wide enough as you jump over so you don't smack your partner in the head with your leg on the way over.) As soon as the jumper lands on his feet (Fig. 23), he turns low, pivots, and scampers behind and then between his partner's legs (Fig. 24). (As you go under, keep your head low. This helps your technique and keeps your partner from getting bumped in the crotch.) Then hustle back to your feet and start all over again (Fig. 25). Try alternating the drill after ten repetitions and go in front of your partner's legs and then through them. Do three sets of ten reps.

For best results, do these drills three times a week, on the days you are not lifting weights. Make sure you are thoroughly warmed up first.

By leaping, cartwheeling, and duck walking, you will not only

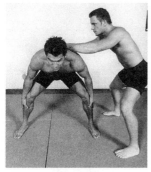

Figure 22

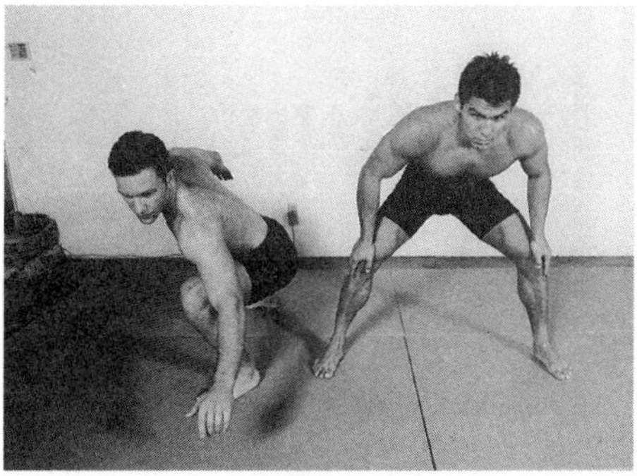

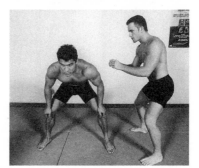

Figure 23

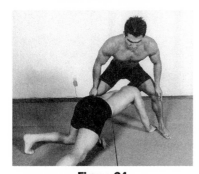

Figure 24

Figure 25

become stronger and more agile, but during real competition you will move with natural instinct, and natural rhythm. In the dog fight that is a scramble, you will prevail.

Chapter 20

Fighting on Your Feet
Strikes, Kicks, and a Devastating Choke

"First we use kicks and strikes to break an opponent's spirit. Then we use submission techniques to finish the fight."

—Guy Mezger, Lion's Den fighter, kickboxing champion, undefeated in the UFC, one of the top-ranked fighters in Pancrase.

T he referee gives the signal and the fight begins. You are on your feet, moving carefully but confidently toward your opponent. What is the best way to attack? In submission fighting, some of your most devastating weapons, or fighting techniques, will come into play on the ground. But you must also be a dangerous striker and kicker. You must be able and willing to fight on your feet for two reasons. First, some fights can be ended on your feet, without going to the ground. Second, you will have much better success shooting in and taking your opponent to the ground after you have landed a combination of strikes and kicks—or at least menaced your opponent with the threat of a solid blow.

Even if you are fighting somebody who is really drunk, a punch or even a fake to the head will help stiffen his body and defenses, making it that much easier to zoom in, shackle his legs, and drop him.

When people shake hands with me, they are often surprised that my hand is not bigger than theirs. But you don't need a huge hand to land a crunching blow. Yes, you do need some strength so your strikes have pop. But just as important, you need timing, control, and finesse. The following is a discussion of several methods of fighting your opponent while on your feet.

The Strike

Let's take a closer look at the strike.

Promoters of the UFC call me a master of submission techniques. While I have studied submission techniques and used them effec-

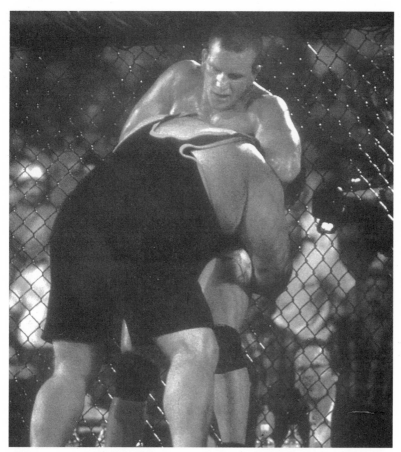

Fighting on your feet means strikes, kicks, and a choke called the guillotine, which Jerry Bohlander used against Scott Ferrozzo in his very first UFC fight.

tively, I have also won several of my UFC and Pancrase matches with strikes. I landed some sharp blows on Royce Gracie in our fight. I was able to strike effectively against Christophe Leininger in UFC III and also against Brian Johnston in the 1996 Ultimate Ultimate.

In bare-knuckle fights, one of the most frequent injuries is a broken hand. It is for this reason that the UFC and other reality fighting events are safer than boxing matches. You don't have the constant pounding of a gloved fist on your face or head. Thus, you don't have the resulting brain damage. When fighting bare-knuckle, if you slam your fist again and again into the head or face of your opponent, all you will do is to fracture your hand. Trust me here. I have done this more than once, most recently in my fight against Brian Johnston.

Most guys who fight bare-knuckle any length of time have broken a hand, or at least some knuckles. But from my point of view, I would rather have a broken hand than a damaged brain.

So when you fight with bare knuckles, or even with a light martial arts glove on, you have to be smart about where, when, and how to strike. You must learn to be surgically precise with your blows. This is done to preserve the condition of your hand, to land the most telling blow, and to preserve your energy. Striking, especially in the supercharged environment of a real fight, takes and uses up a tremendous amount of energy. If you start windmilling or trying to launch haymaker after haymaker, you will be out of gas in short order.

Though I used a light martial arts glove in my Ultimate Ultimate fight against Johnston, I do not believe I will use them again. A bare knuckle used precisely can do more damage and bring a quicker tap-out than a fist enclosed in even a light glove.

When you strike with bare knuckles, you should make contact with the full front of your fist, not with a single knuckle. This method will both help to protect your knuckles and allow your hand to better absorb the shock of the blow. There is an exception, however. When you are in your opponent's guard, that is, you are on top of him and his legs are around your waist, you can deliver painful jabs to your opponent's ribs using your knuckles. Try to find a rib that is most exposed, the most bony, or aim for the lowest rib, which is usually the

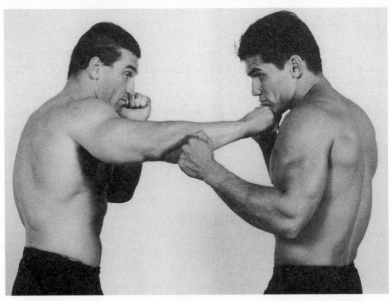

Figure 1

smallest and weakest. Then, jab away using short strikes, and digging your knuckle into the rib cage. You can do this because the ribs are not as hard as the skull or forehead, and your blows from this position are short and controlled, but with enough power to damage and wear down your opponent without shattering your knuckle.

For stand-up attacks, I tell my fighters there is a strike zone they must aim their attacks within. The strike zone runs from the base of your opponent's chin to the bridge of his nose, and from cheekbone to cheekbone. This is an area with some bone but with some soft tissue and cartilage. Striking within this area will usually do damage to your opponent, without damaging your own hand. You can split a lip, break a nose, raise a welt or cut under an eye. Moreover, if you strike the chin properly, you can drop an opponent instantly.

Some guys just strike blindly, even with closed eyes. Needless to say, that method doesn't work very well. When I throw a punch I aim it, just like you would aim a rifle or an arrow. I usually aim a punch for the base of the chin (Fig. 1). If I hit the bull's eye, I am able to stun or knock out my opponent. If he lowers his chin, I strike his nose; if he raises it, I can strike his throat or his chest. If I am striking from the guard or the mount position (when you are mounted, you are on top of your opponent, on his chest, and his legs are behind you), I usually punch at the center of the nose, since there is less distance to close and less chance of his head moving too far out of the strike zone. When you mount them, most guys will try to cover or turn their faces away. When that happens, you can punch the ears or go for the tip of the jaw. Eventually, if you persist, they will cover the ear or jaw, or shift position, and expose the strike zone again.

If you have ever boxed and then tried bare-knuckle fighting, you have probably found yourself throwing a lot of punches that miss their intended target. This simply happens because your fist is less than half the size of a typical boxing glove. You must be considerably quicker and more accurate to land a blow with your bare fist than with a gloved fist. In other words, your strikes must become swift and crisp.

If you wind-up for a haymaker, unless you are awfully good or lucky, all you will hit is air. Instead, strike quickly with a compact wind-up. If your punch is precise, it can do plenty of damage without rearing back like Popeye does. It is a little like hitting a home run; you don't have to hit the ball extremely hard to send it, you just have to hit it right. This might sound basic, but you would be surprised at how many guys don't follow the basic premise of a punch: keeping your eyes open and focused on the target.

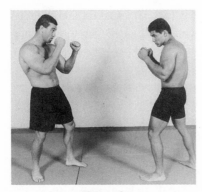

Figure 2

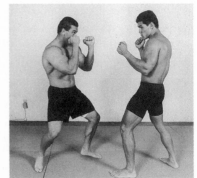

Figure 3

To develop deep punching penetration, use a heavy punching bag. As you practice striking a punching bag, try to get a snap into the blow. The fist should zing to its target, then zing back to defend against an incoming blow or to prepare for another attack. As you punch, make sure you keep your other hand up and near your chin for defense. Otherwise, as you punch, your opponent will too, and he might have a better chance of connecting than you.

Another reason to keep your punches quick and compact is that if you extend too far or too slowly, you will open yourself up to being taken down. Instead of overextending your arm to hit a target, close the distance with your feet (Figs. 2, 3). Practice stepping in as you throw a punch. Take a step closer to your opponent, making sure that you are in balance and your hands are up, and then punch. Practice moving toward a bag and throwing a series of punches. Another way is to practice with a partner, pulling the punch, or striking a focus mitt as you step forward. These drills will help.you to gauge distances and striking angles, and give you a better hit-to-miss ratio.

My fighters often ask me about body blows. I don't use them much while I'm fighting on my feet. In a bare-knuckle match, if you are close enough to land a body blow, you are close enough to go for the strike zone and do much more damage. You are also close enough to take your opponent down and finish with a submission.

Once you are within striking distance, set up the finishing punch with a jab, or a series of jabs. The jab is usually agitating to an opponent, not a finishing blow. You probe with a jab, get your opponent off guard, then follow with a strong punch. While a jab is not typically decisive, it can be very effective. Land enough jabs and you can bloody and frustrate an opponent.

If your opponent shoots in on you, my general rule is this: don't strike. You have to get too low to land an uppercut, one of the only striking defenses against this type of attack. If you strike, you will only hit the top or side of your opponent's head and risk injury to yourself. It is okay to land a palm strike to either ear, though. Otherwise, it is better to either raise a knee into your opponent's incoming face or sprawl on top of him to gain the superior position. I will discuss the sprawl in more detail later.

The Guillotine

If your opponent is charging at you to shoot and take you down, there is another option: go for a guillotine choke. This is not an easy movement, but, if mastered, it can be devastating. You can use it when your opponent comes in with his head down, instead of up, as you want your opponent's head on your hip for this technique (Fig. 4). Spread and bend your legs to keep your balance. Drop your legs back on the side you are applying the guillotine. Looping your arm around your opponent's head, keeping it low (Fig. 5). After you loop your arm around your opponent's neck, grasp your opposite arm, tightly then cinch the choke.

With the guillotine (and this applies to other chokes as well) turn your arm so the bony side is facing up as you choke. You want the arm to act like a knife blade, slipping deep into your opponent's neck and

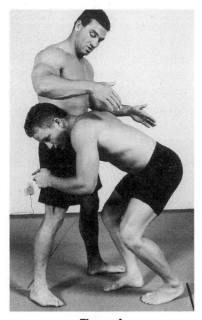

Figure 4

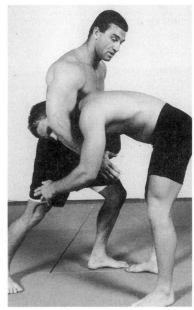

Figure 5

exerting maximum pressure and pain. If you can, work the choke so that it is applied by the portion of your forearm closest to your wrist. This is the narrowest, boniest part of your arm—the sharpest part of the blade.

Please keep in mind, however, that you must do all of this rather quickly, while making sure your opponent can't slip a hand in to buffer the choke and make it ineffective. Once you have the choke hold set, rock back, arching your back, and cinch even tighter. Try to lodge your choking arm across your opponent's Adam's apple. This will cause excruciating pain. The guillotine is the technique I used to defeat Dan Severn in our first Superfight. Severn came in low with his head down to grab one of my legs. I quickly looped his neck and cinched it up. He was forced to tap out. In addition, Jerry Bohlander, one of the Lion's Den fighters, used a guillotine to subdue Scott Ferrozzo in their UFC VIII fight in Puerto Rico.

Get a good guillotine sunk in, and your opponent is finished. His head is down, he is probably disoriented, his oxygen is being cut off, he may feel his Adam's apple being crushed, and if he tries to shift his weight, he only adds more pressure to the choke.

The Crucifix

At the Lion's den, we are constantly experimenting with new moves. As I mentioned earlier, submission fighting is always changing, always evolving, always progressing. One move that has evolved at Lion's Den is called the crucifix. While I don't know of any other dojo that uses this technique, I am not claiming that we invented it, either. Chances are good that a crafty Greek pancration fighter used the technique a thousand years ago. The crucifix is an effective submission move, one that involves the classic submission blend of speed and strength. The crucifix can either be applied during a clinch or when your opponent tries to shoot in on you. It was used by Jerry Bohlander in dramatic fashion in UFC VII to win the Lightweight Championship.

To perform this technique, place one of your arms under your opponent's armpits and press your hand into his back (Fig. 6). (This move is called an underhook.) With your head firmly planted against your opponent's back, place your free arm over your opponent's other arm, wrapping it around the arm tightly (Fig. 7). (This move is called an overhook.) As long as your weight is above your opponent's, and his head is locked under you, you should now be able to control and move your opponent. Keeping your feet wide and maintaining your balance, shift your hips and torque your opponent to the mat, driving him to a

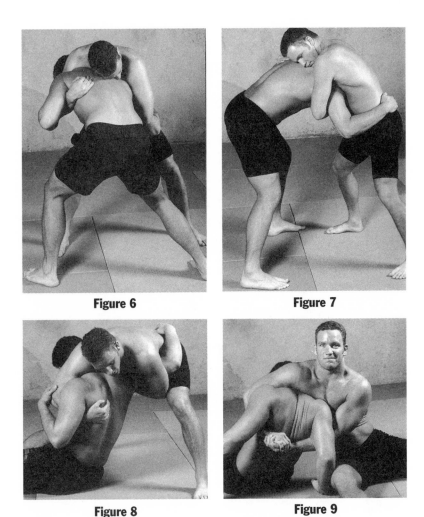

Figure 6

Figure 7

Figure 8

Figure 9

sitting position (Fig. 8). Now, quickly switch the arm that is overhooking your opponent to an underhook, so that you can clasp your hands behind your opponent's back. This must be done quickly, otherwise your opponent may turn and break free from the hold. At this point, if you have achieved a solid double underhook, his neck should be below your armpit (Fig. 9). Now squeeze your hands together tightly, putting pressure on his shoulders and neck, and causing a great deal of pain.

Opponents who will not tap out immediately will do so eventually, as the crucifix steadily cuts off the flow of air to the brain. The main point is to keep tightening your hands and arms into a kind of noose, while pressing down on the back of your opponent's neck.

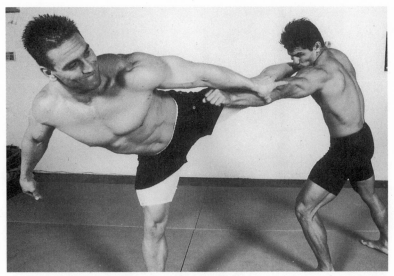

Figure 10

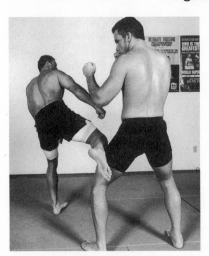

Figure 11

Kicking

Now let's talk about kicks. In the UFC, I wear wrestling shoes so I can get better traction on the canvas, move faster, and draw more power from my lower body. Because I wear shoes, UFC rules prevent me from kicking. Even so, kicks are an important part of the Lion's Den fighter's arsenal.

Think about this: a kick can deliver more of a wallop than a punch, in addition to covering a much longer distance. Try standing straight and reach out with your arm. How far can you reach? Now extend your leg and stretch out your foot. If you are like most guys, the reach with your foot is at least fifteen inches longer than the reach with your fist (Fig. 10). As a result, a kick can be a devastating long-distance attack.

Kicks can be delivered like jabs or punches. Repeated jab-like kicks to the thigh (Fig. 11) or ribs can steadily weaken an opponent, setting him up for a big kick to the neck or head, or a punch or submission hold.

Remember this: No matter what, do not kick with your foot. The proper way is to kick with the lower part of your shin. There are dozens of bones in your foot, many of them very fragile. If you slam your foot against somebody's head or knee, you may fracture it in many places. Your shin, on the other hand, is a thick, heavy bone. It might get bruised and bloody, but it will probably not break.

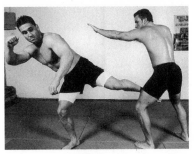

When you kick, keep your legs bent and flexible. A kick is executed in a fluid motion that uses the momentum created by your hips. A key to a quick and accurate kick is a sharp pivot on your supporting foot, as if you were getting ready to kick a soc-

Figure 12

cer ball (Fig. 12). Think about a field-goal kicker in football. Notice how his knees are bent, how he swings his hips through the motion, how he pivots and always keeps his eye on the target. In a tighter, faster sequence, those are the elements of a good martial arts kick.

An excellent tactic when street fighting is to set up a kick with a punch or a feint to your opponent's face. Your opponent will almost always bring his hands up to protect himself, which leaves him vulnerable to a blow from below. A good kick to the thigh can force your opponent to drop to the ground or stumble, giving you a quick advantage. If you land enough kicks to the thighs, your opponent will naturally drop his hands to defend his aching legs. Then, whoosh, you can swing around with a kick to the neck and head (Fig. 13).

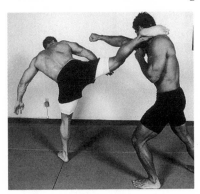

Figure 13

We do not practice low sweeps to the ankle or lower leg. You will probably miss the target with these techniques because your opponent only has to move a few inches to avoid the attack. And if you don't miss, you will likely hit your opponent's ankle, shin, or knee, which can hurt you as much if not more than it does your opponent.

At the Lion's Den we bring in martial artists from various disciplines to help us grow and learn. In return, if we can help them with grappling or submission techniques, we do. One of the best martial artists we have had work with us is world kickboxing champion Maurice Smith. Maurice showed us how devastating kicks can be during his October, 1996 Extreme Fighting bout against defending heavyweight champion Conan Silviera. Maurice pounded on Silviera's legs, punishing Silviera and forcing him to drop his hands. At this, Smith launched a roundhouse kick to Silviera's head and neck. That kick was one of the most spectacular I have seen in any fight. It struck like lightning, sending Silviera tumbling to the ropes, dazed and defeated.

But Maurice did not try to win the fight in the opening seconds with a big kick. He took his time, wearing Silveira down, landing kick after kick on Silveira's thighs. It was like chopping down a tree. I tell all my fighters to go first for the thighs. If you land a good kick to the thigh, it can almost paralyze the muscles and will cause extreme pain. Your opponent will be wounded, physically and mentally.

It should be noted that Maurice did not walk into that fight with only kicking and striking skills. Maurice has learned grappling and submission skills too, and those skills allowed him to fight effectively against Silviera when they went to the ground.

Kicks can be especially potent late in a fight, when your opponent is too tired to move out of the way or defend himself effectively. An example of a great kicking assault was seen in UFC VII, when Marco Ruas destroyed Paul Varelans with repeated kicks to the thighs. Varelans, who is a good man and a fine fighter, could have defended himself against those kicks fairly simply by raising his attacked leg and bending it, deflecting the kick off your right knee or shin. Again, if he strikes your knee or shin, it will most likely hurt him more than it will hurt you.

I mentioned earlier that the shinbone is pretty solid and seldom breaks. But I do know of fighters who have actually splintered their shinbones by kicking the knee. As a result, unlike muay Thai training in Thailand, we practice our kicks against a heavy bag, focus mitts, and through light sparring.

I also teach my fighters to defend themselves against a vari-

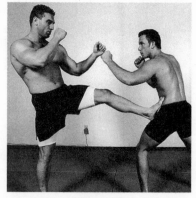

Figure 14

ety of kicks and strikes with what we call a hip check (Fig. 14). This is a simple move which, unlike a kick, uses the foot instead of the shin to make contact. It is a quick blow to the opponent's incoming hip that can derail a strike and throw a kick off target. It is a defensive movement, but it can frustrate your opponent and allow you to set up a kick or a strike of your own. It can also help you gauge the distance between you and your opponent.

The Shoot

Once you have punched and kicked and softened up your opponent, or see an opening to take him to the ground, you are ready for the shoot. The shoot is a quick, explosive movement that uses your weight to drive your opponent to the ground. It is critical in submission fighting.

As you shoot, be sure to aim and keep your body low and to penetrate through your opponent. When I tutor Lion's Den fighters on the shoot, I tell them to think about driving their opponent through an imaginary window. To do this, you need to gain momentum and to control your opponent's lower body to lift and dump him to the ground.

When do you shoot? The basic shoot can come when your opponent tries to punch or kick you. Basically, you can shoot any time your opponent is in motion and his balance is shifting. Moreover, you can set up a shoot by moving to your opponent's side. As he turns to square up to you, bam—you shoot in.

Start the basic shoot by bending your knees and getting low, really low (Fig. 15). Remember the duck walk. As you drop, keep your face up so you do not get guillotined. Bring your hands out in front of you to protect your face, almost like you are ready to dive (Fig. 16). All this is done as you move toward your opponent, thrusting your shoulder into his knee closest to you (Fig. 17). Drive your shoulder through that knee toward his other knee, in effect smashing your opponent's legs together. As you do this, wrap your arms around the legs, tighten them like a noose, and your opponent should drop like a stone (Figs. 18, 19). Make sure to keep your hands up to shield your face in case your opponent raises a knee as you move toward him.

Make sure you don't drop to your own knees until your opponent is on his way down. If you have ever played football, driving through your man was probably part of your basic tackling instruction. Again, I want to stress that you do not go to your knees until you have finished the shoot and your opponent is going down. Otherwise, your opponent may escape and hit you with a kick, or

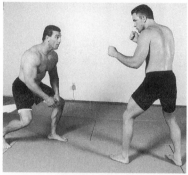

Figure 15

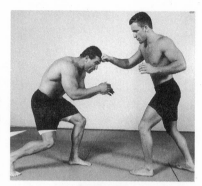

Figure 16

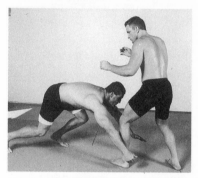

Figure 17

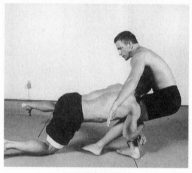

Figure 18

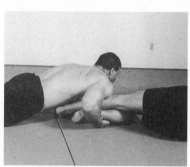

Figure 19

slip behind you and apply a choke hold.

To shoot in off a kick, block the kick using your arms and hands and spin your opponent's legs to the side (Fig. 20). Then, drop and shoot through your opponent from behind. Drive your shoulder into the back of your opponent's knees as described above (Fig. 21). If all goes well, your opponent will land hard on his stomach, and you will be on top of him, in a perfect position for a rear choke.

To shoot off a punch, drop low as your opponent swings at you (Fig. 22). If he wants to throw a punch, your opponent has to post, or place his weight, on his lead leg. Go for that leg, staying low to avoid the punch. Drive your shoulder into and through his back knee, wrap the legs, and put him down.

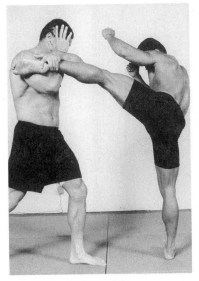

Figure 20

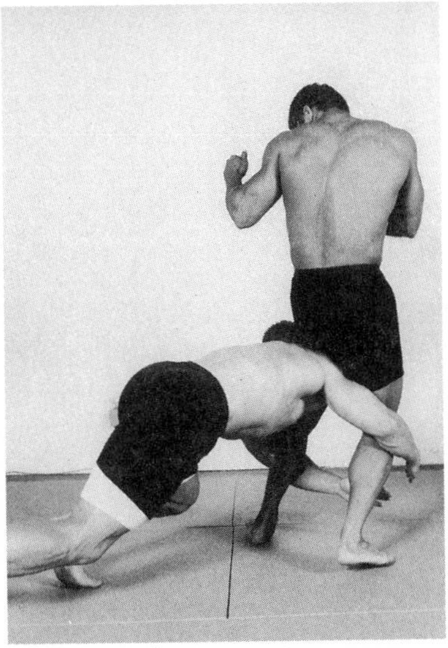

Figure 21

Done right, the shoot is one of the most explosive movements in the martial arts. A good shooter can close the distance and take his opponent down in less than two seconds, gaining an important advantage.

The Sprawl

If you your opponent keeps his head down and you can get a guillotine, fine.

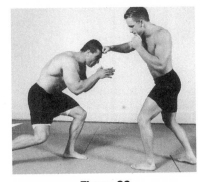

Figure 22

More often, the most effective way to defend against a shoot is by sprawling. The sprawl will put you on top of your opponent and turn the fight to your advantage.

This is how the sprawl works. As your opponent shoots, get your hips and legs back and tilt your weight over your opponent's neck and shoulders (Fig. 23). It's very important to keep your legs back and away from your opponent because he is probably trying to grab a leg and take you down. You can sprawl and stop a man by putting your hands outside of his arms, but that's not the best way. It's more effective to wedge your arm and shoulder between his arm and head (Fig. 24). This stops his progress more efficiently. As the sprawl progresses,

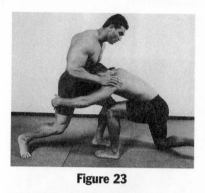

Figure 23

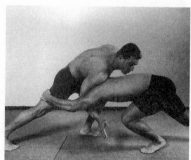

Figure 24

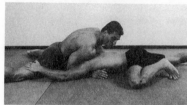

Figure 25

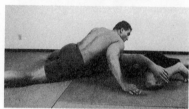

Figure 26

you place your sternum over your opponent's neck and drive him down. As you do this, spread your legs and continue to keep them, away from your opponent's hands. The idea is to smash him to the ground or mat, with you on top (Fig. 25). This will not only leave you in the controlling position, it should stun him and give you a quick psychological advantage. Now you should be in a good position to go for a choke or armbar (Fig. 26).

So you have tenderized your opponent with strikes and kicks and taken him down with a quick, clean shoot or sprawl. The end may be very near.

Let's talk ground submissions.

Chapter 21

Control

Building the Foundation

"What is submissions? That's simple. Submissions is what works."

—Vernon White, Lion's Den fighter and Pancrase veteran
with a background in taekwondo.

I f your fight goes to the ground, you can start moving toward applying one of many choke or submission holds. In most cases, however, you will need to achieve a position of transitional control before attempting your finishing submission move.

To master submission techniques, or even gain a good grasp of it, you must learn the basics. At the Lion's Den, this knowledge is gained

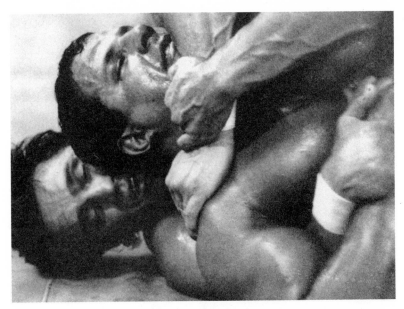

Mike Radnov, one of my training partners, is a big, strong guy. But if you master the control positions of submissions, you can dominate even much larger opponents.

through an understanding of the ten control positions of submissions, inside and out. These ten positions are the platforms from which you will launch your submissions attacks. The purpose of the positions is to gain control of your opponent and then exert enough pressure or pain on your opponent so that he will move and reveal an opening, allowing you go for the finishing move.

From these positions, you can achieve either chokes, leg submissions, armbars, or you can launch a final barrage of strikes. If you learn these ten positions well, the submission techniques that follow will flow naturally, automatically. Again, the fight is in the preparation. Basics are absolutely critical to your preparation for combat. Let's now go through the ten control positions of submission techniques.

Position 1, The Head Vice

To assume the head vice position (Fig. 1), keep your legs spread, extending one and bending the other at the knee. It is important to keep your center of gravity below that of your opponent. To do this, keep your sternum slightly lower than your opponents and bury your weight

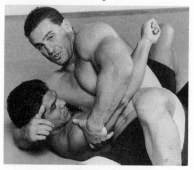

Figure 1

into his chest, with one arm locked tightly around his neck, the other controlling his arm at the triceps. Keep his head elevated off the mat—this will prevent him from bridging or arching up and rolling out of the hold. Trap his arm tightly behind the triceps by pulling it off the mat into your chest so that he cannot push you away or punch you. Your opponent will have a hard time breathing in this position. His neck will also become uncomfortable because you are torquing his head. From the head vice position, you can move to applying a

choke hold or an armbar.

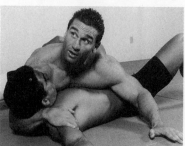

Figure 2

Position 2, The Side Mount

To assume the side mount position (Fig. 2), spread your legs until they are flat in a straddle position, and your weight is pressed into your opponent's chest. Again, keep your center of gravity low and make sure you do not arch too high in order to achieve control. If you rise too high, you will be vulnerable to being rolled over by your opponent. Keep one arm around your opponent's neck and force it off the mat to prevent him from bridging, and clamp your other around his triceps. As with position one, a choke hold or an armbar are techniques which can be launched naturally from this platform.

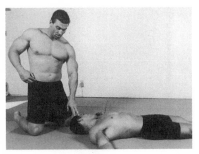

Figure 3

Position 3, The Hip Grinder

To employ the hip grinder (Figs. 3, 4), slide onto your opponent from above, moving your

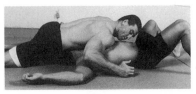

Figure 4

hipbone into his temple. This causes substantial pain and forces him to move, thus provide you with an opening. As with position two, spread your legs in the straddle position for balance. To secure the position, you must control your opponent's arms. Assuming you are using your right hipbone and moving it into your opponent's right temple, you will wrap your left arm around his left arm from the outside, clamp it tight, and tuck your head down toward your fist. Next, hook your right arm around his right arm from inside, inserting your hand between his ribs and triceps. As you achieve balance, your opponent will move because the hip causes a lot of pain. When he moves you can pursue a submission hold.

Position 4, The Mount, Legs Tucked Under

The mount is a dominant position to either launch strikes or move

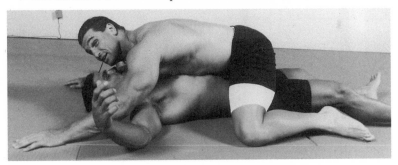

Figure 5

into a submission technique. In the mount position (Fig. 5), it is important to control your opponent's legs. Otherwise, you could be pushed or lifted off of your opponent. Begin position four with your knees planted outside of your opponent's hips, with your feet flat against the mat. Slip your feet next to your opponent's legs. Move your arms out wide and plant them on the mat outside your opponent's shoulders and put your weight into your opponent's chest. Again, he will have difficulty breathing and you will have achieved a dominant position of control. From this position, you can safely execute a series of strikes with fist or elbows, or you can move to various arm or leg submission holds.

Position 5, The Mount, Legs Tucked Over

This is similar to position four, except you tuck your legs over your opponent's legs, pressing much of your weight into his thighs and digging your feet in,

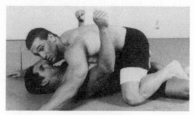

Figure 6

just above his knees (Fig. 6). Again, keep your hands out so your opponent can not roll you over. From this mount position, you may launch strikes leading to transitional movements to finally apply an effective leg submission hold.

Position 6, Leg Clamp

Position six is actually a transitional movement from position 5 described above (Fig. 7). Unlike the other basic positions, however, this one is not used for control; it is in fact a direct move into any number of submission techniques, including an ankle lock, toe hold,

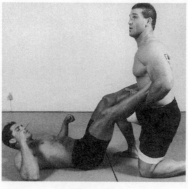

Figure 7

or kneebar. To achieve the leg clamp position, swing back from your mount position and lock your opponent's legs under your armpits. Dig the bones of your forearms into your opponent's Achilles and press them tightly. One or both of your knees may be on the mat. The only way for your opponent to try and escape from this position is to roll. When he does, he becomes vulnerable and

you can shift to a finishing submission hold.

Position 7, Back Mount, Legs Under

The back mount is an excellent position because you can
either move to a choke hold or

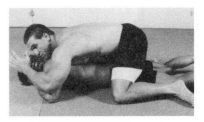

Figure 8

armbar or punish your opponent with blows to the face, neck, or ears
(Fig. 8). Keep your knees and legs outside of your opponent's thighs
and flat on the canvas, but be prepared to slip them under your opponent's legs if he tries to roll or raise to his knees. Press your chest into
his back and spread your arms out to the mat for maximum control.

Position 8, Back Mount, Legs Over

Position eight is very similar
to position seven. In this position,
it is important to keep your legs
on top of your opponent's legs
(Fig. 9). Lock your feet between

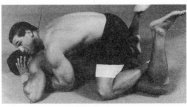

Figure 9

your opponent's knees. Then use your feet and legs to spread his legs
apart. He will then have no base of power or balance. From this position, you can control your opponent while working toward a rear choke.

Position 9, Back Side Mount

To assume the back side mount, spread your legs for balance and
keep your center of gravity low (Fig. 10). Wrap your arm around his

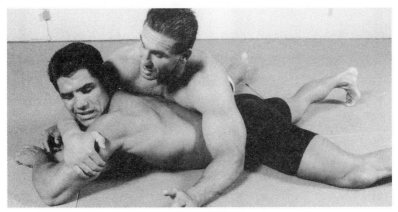

Figure 10

head and shoulder. Bring your other arm around and pin your elbow into his hips to help control his lower body. This gives you good control and can lead to a back or side choke.

Position 10, Nose Grinder

To assume this position, move your chest over the back of your opponent. Your ribcage is on the back of his head (Fig. 11). Keep your legs spread for balance. Grab his arms and hook under his elbows, keeping them off the mat. If you control his elbows, he can't roll. Because

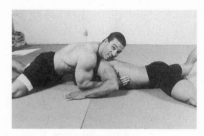

Figure 11

your weight is on his head, he cannot bridge. He also feels like he is being slowly smothered, his face being ground into the mat. So he will wriggle, opening himself up to a choke or submission hold.

Chapter 22

Ground Attack

Chokes, Arm and Leg Submissions

"When you get a good choke or submission hold, it's over. It's as simple as that."

—Tra Telligman, Lion's Den fighter and
Hawaiian Superbrawl super heavyweight champion

You are on the ground and you have moved to a controlling position. From here, you want to finish the fight quickly and victoriously. You can finish with strikes, but if your opponent is skilled that can take a long time and your hand might ache for weeks afterward.

If possible, you want to go for a choke or a submission hold that will exert pressure on your opponent's arm, leg, Achilles tendon, or

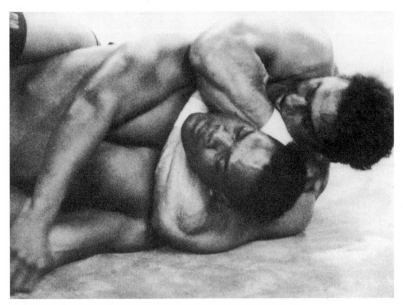

In the Lion's Den, if you make a mistake, you may be choked out. Here Vernon White is the victim of a rear choke administered by yours truly.

ankle, forcing him to tap out. Most choke and submission holds work quickly. While many street fighters and even martial artists are familiar with delivering strikes and kicks while standing, relatively few know much about chokes or submission techniques.

Chokes

If you learn and perfect enough chokes, you will get a feel for them and your opponent's weak points. You can feel for the Adam's apple, feel for the veins, feel for the windpipe. With a choke, you either want to close off the supply of blood or air, or put enough pressure on the Adam's apple to cause sufficient pain for a tap out. You learned the guillotine as part of the section on stand-up fighting, so let's move on to some other chokes here.

The Rear Choke

The rear choke (Fig. 1) is a common and very effective technique, and can be achieved from control positions seven and eight. Before you apply the rear choke, dig your legs under your opponent so he can't thrash and slip away from you. Plant your chest firmly into your opponent's back and wrap your forearm around his neck. Slip your fingers

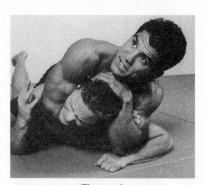

Figure 1

through and clamp·them into your biceps. As with a guillotine, you want to use the edge of your wrist to dig into your opponent's neck. As you are setting the choke, push your free hand on the top of your opponent's head and press down. For added force, use your own head to press down, thus maximizing the downward pressure.

Once you have the choke cinched up (i.e., tight), pull the elbow of your choking arm up and back, cranking your opponent's neck. In this way, much of the force of the choke is accomplished with the large muscles of your back and shoulder, not your arm. You can finish a rear choke with only your arm muscles, but this method can greatly tire those muscles, especially if your opponent has a neck like a bull. Done correctly, this approach creates a triple whammy: 1) air and blood is blocked with the upward force of your wrist bone (or you have painful pressure on the Adam's apple), 2) your free hand and head are pressing down, further constricting air and blood flow, and

3) your back and shoulder muscles are torquing the neck.

Some points on the rear choke to keep in mind: If your opponent digs his chin into his chest to block a choke, be patient. Try using a cross-face with your free fist and forearm, by scraping across his mouth and nose. Other methods include striking his nose to get him to raise his jaw, striking the back of his head or his ear with an elbow strike, or just going ahead and cinching the jaw. This will cause enough discomfort that your opponent will probably shift position, allowing penetration to his neck.

The Leg Choke

A leg choke is typically done when your opponent is in your guard. The key is to get one leg up and around your opponent's neck, with his arm kept outside that leg (Fig. 2). You do this by grabbing one of his hands and pushing it back, while raising your knee along the same arm. Bring the knee up to his ear and swing your lower leg and foot behind his back. After that, lock the foot of the leg under the knee of your free leg, which will keep your opponent from going anywhere. Next, shove your opponent's free arm under his chin, while clamping legs around his neck (Fig. 3). Once opponent's arm is across and more or less out of the way, grab your his head with both hands and pull it down (Fig. 4). Now, squeeze your legs tighter and tighter as you hold the head down, and rock your hips gradually to the side. If your opponent succeeds in rolling you

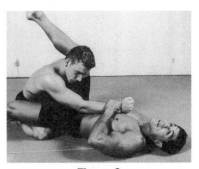

Figure 2

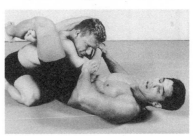

Figure 3

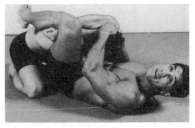

Figure 4

over without tapping, just hang on. Pretty soon you will be on top of him, and your legs will still be around his neck, tighter than ever. If need be, you can deliver some strikes to speed things along.

Knowing he's trapped and virtually immobile, your opponent may either tap out quickly, or hang on and attempt a roll. The constriction of blood and air during this technique is not as rapid as it is with the rear choke. However, as with most choke holds, be patient. The critical part of the leg choke is getting that one leg up and around your opponent's neck and getting his arm on the outside of your leg. Once that leg is firmly locked with your other leg, your opponent is on his way to tapping out.

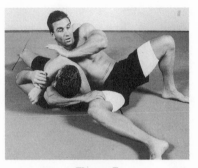

Figure 5

The Side Choke

Like the rear choke, the side choke is a relatively quick finishing move. A warning though: as you do the side choke, do not allow your opponent to duck his head, slip the choke, and move behind you. If he does, he'll be in a good position to apply a rear choke, and you may be the one tapping out.

To begin the side choke, slip your arm under the back of your

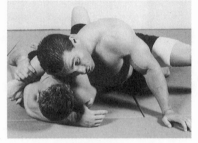

Figure 6

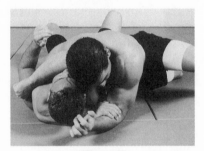

Figure 7

opponent's neck (Fig. 5). His arm and elbow closest to you is free and can be dangerous, so check the elbow with your hand as you perform a hip-heist, a wrestling move in which you sweep your legs under and behind you (Fig. 6). Spread your legs for good stability and then grab your free forearm with the hand of the arm you are choking with (Fig. 7). Move your neck against his triceps, both to control it and to help apply choking pressure. Most of the pressure is exerted against the side of your opponent's neck, cutting off the flow of blood.

In my very first match for Pancrase, I used a side choke on Masa Funaki, forcing him to tap out. The side choke is a reliable and efficient part of the submissions arsenal.

Armbars

Both arm and leg submissions share one thing: you must control the limb being submitted with both legs. Again, that is why leg strength is so important in our submissions fighting system. You will use your legs to capture another fighter's arm or leg and clamp it firmly. With this kind of control, the limb may be bent to the point where your opponent must either tap out or suffer damage to his joint.

Keep in mind that once you have secured an arm or leg, it only takes an inch or less of movement to create substantial pain and, in most cases, a tap out. Once the limb is cinched tightly, the actual submission pressure should be exerted smoothly and with a controlled motion. You do not want to waste valuable time and energy achieving control of an arm or leg just to lose the hold as you apply the finishing force.

I must stress that as you go for a submission, expect to get hit or kicked once or twice before your opponent finally taps out. I got kicked by Pat Smith in the first UFC as I applied a heel hook. I got headbutted by Kimo Leopoldo in my Superfight in Puerto Rico before I could force him to tap out with a knee bar. While you will likely be challenged as you apply a submission hold, do not give up. If you are prepared and tenacious, your hold will do the job intended and you will prevail.

With armbars, pressure is exerted on the elbow joint. To effect an armbar, you must control your opponent's arm with your own arms and hands, then wedge it tightly between your thighs. You then crank the arm backward, putting great pressure on the elbow joint. The leverage point is between your thighs, held tightly enough so your opponent's arm will not slip out.

Escape and Armbar

You can quickly move from a vulnerable position below your opponent to a controlling position with an armbar in place. For purposes of illustration, we will assume you are going for your opponent's left arm. First grip your opponent's hand and hold it to your chest (Fig. 8). Next, swing your legs up to your chest, keeping one knee against your oppo-

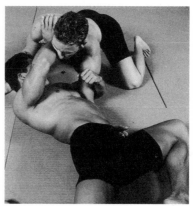

Figure 8

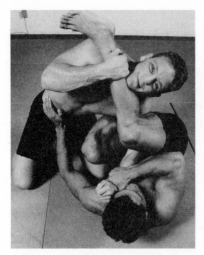

Figure 9

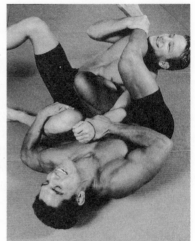

Figure 10

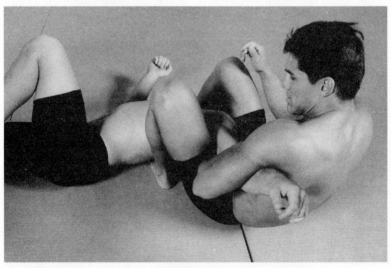

Figure 11

nent's ribs and extending the other leg up and around his neck (Fig. 9). Quickly push his head down with the leg as you rock forward, while maintaining control of the arm to be pressured (Fig. 10). Slip your forearm below your opponent's elbow, lock his forearm under your armpit, and slowly rock back, making sure your feet and thighs are clamping tightly (Fig. 11). Make sure, too, that your right leg remains over your opponent's neck. Otherwise, he can roll over your legs and strike you.

Armbar from Guard

An armbar is a good technique when you have your opponent in your guard. It's key that you have your opponent high in your chest, so you can control him; if he's well down on your ribcage, an armbar is difficult to accomplish. Let's assume that you are going for his left arm. First, grip his left wrist with your right arm (Fig. 12). At the same time, slip your left hand under his knee. This helps control his leg and prevents him from kneeing or kicking you. It also helps move you in position to bring your right leg up and trap his head. Be aware that during this move, you may be vulnerable to a strike with his right hand. So move fast. Push his head down as you tighten your grip on

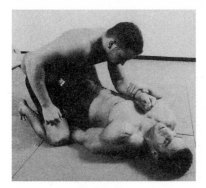

Figure 12

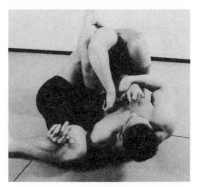

Figure 13

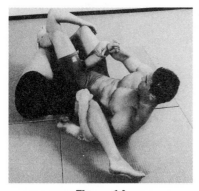

Figure 14

his left arm between your legs and continue to control his right leg (Fig. 13). Now comes the fun part. With his arm now between your legs, acting as a vice, pull his arm down toward your belly (Fig. 14). If you have the arm firmly pinched between your legs, it takes very little downward bend to create intense pain and a tap-out. Raise your shoulder up to give you better leverage.

Rear Mount Armbar

When you have a rear mount, your first option is to apply a choke hold. However, if your opponent is using his hands to effectively check your choke you can go for an armbar as it fast and not too complicated. To apply the rear mount armbar, slip your left arm around

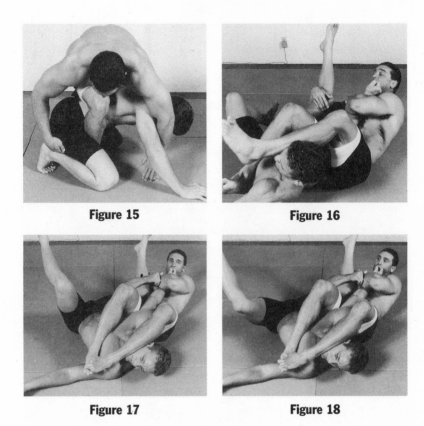

Figure 15

Figure 16

Figure 17

Figure 18

your opponent's right upper arm and slip your right arm around his right thigh (Fig. 15). Now roll forward, at the same time flipping your opponent (Fig. 16). As you come out of the roll, cinch both his leg and arm toward your chest (Fig. 17). Make sure your feet are pressing down on his neck and shoulder. In this position he can't move, and you have dominant leverage on his arm. Rock back slowly, and your opponent will either tap out or injure his arm (Fig. 18).

Armbar off the Hammer Lock

This move illustrates how most armbars develop. You will not usually be lucky enough to simply grasp an outstretched hand, clamp the arm between your legs, and rock back—it takes a little time, a little finesse. The technique begins by first grasping a fist or a bent arm, gaining leverage with your legs, then extending that arm so it is reasonably straight and can be bent to a point of tremendous pain. By applying an armbar off the hammer lock, you are able to control your opponent's bent arm.

To perform this technique, grasp your wrist, making sure the edge of your forearm is placed next your opponent's inner elbow (Figs. 19, 20). Then, sit back using the edge of your forearm to put pressure on your opponent's arm so that it straightens (Fig. 21). Keep one leg across your opponent's neck and the other wedged against the middle of his back for balance. To finish, rock back slowly and surely, being careful to maintain a strong grip on your opponent's arm (Fig. 22).

Leg Submissions

I want to go over the essentials again before we proceed with leg submissions. It is essential that you wrap both of your legs around one of your opponent's legs to achieve a submission; one leg and one arm is simply not enough. Both of your legs are needed to control one of your opponent's legs—no exceptions. In most cases, you will lock the leg between your thighs just above your crotch. If you try to lock the leg between your knees instead of the strongest, deepest part of your thighs, your opponent can spin out. You must be prepared for a kick or strike as you apply your submission hold. That is another reason

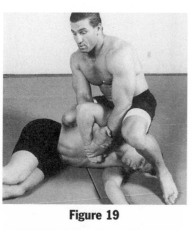

Figure 19

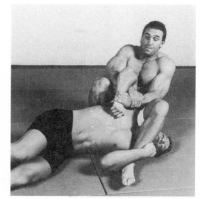

Figure 20

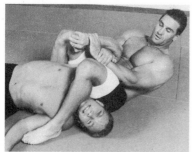

Figure 21

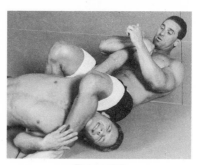

Figure 22

you should soften up your opponent with strikes or kicks early on in a fight. A flurry of kicks or strikes sets up a submissions technique quite effectively because you have achieved an element of surprise. Again, you must be well-rounded. You must have a variety of weapons to use against your opponent, to keep him off-balance, to surprise him, to forcefully seize whatever opportunity that may arise.

Kneebar from the Side Mount

I used the kneebar from the sidemount technique in one of my Pancrase matches to force Bas Rutten, a fine fighter from Holland, to tap out. To apply this technique, you must quickly rise above your opponent and whip a leg over his chest and around one of his legs, trapping his knee in your elbow (Figs. 23, 24). Now you are straddling his leg. Secure your grip with both hands, one pinning the back of his knee, the other his foot. Next, sit back on your opponent's chest, keeping his leg close to your body (Fig. 25). By sitting on his chest, you will knock the air out of your opponent while at the same time stretching the tendons of his knee to the point of submission. As you stretch his leg, gravity and positioning will cause you to roll off his chest. As you do, arch your back to exert maximum pressure on his knee (Fig. 26).

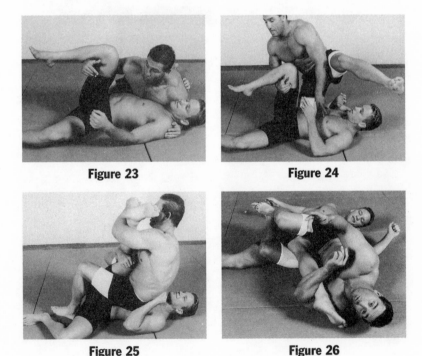

Figure 23   Figure 24

Figure 25   Figure 26

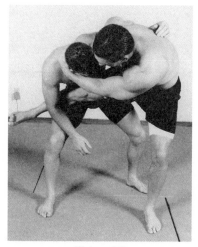

Figure 27

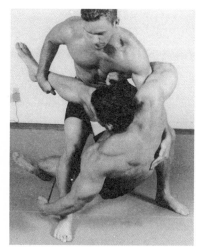

Figure 28

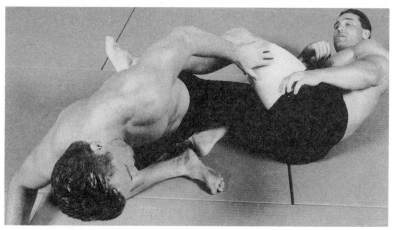

Figure 29

Takedown and Leg Submission

You can employ the takedown and leg submission combination from a standing position where you and your opponent are "locked-up" together. To do this, swing one leg over your opponent's thigh (Fig. 27). His natural reaction will be to trap it, which is fine. Slip your other leg between his legs while simultaneously trapping the back of his heel with your hand as you go down (Fig. 28). He will drop beside you, and you will have control of his leg. Clinch your legs together, pop his foot under your armpit, with one forearm securing it from below, and rock back (Fig. 29).

Kneebar off the Guard

This is a variation of the hold I used against Kimo Leopoldo in our Superfight in Puerto Rico. As with most submission holds, you should go for the move only after you have had a chance to wear down your opponent for a time, dulling his alertness so you can strike quickly and decisively. This move can be used from the full guard if your opponent tries to rear back and get a better distance from which to throw punches, like Kimo did. It can also be used from the half guard, when one of your opponent's legs is outside of your legs. (In the full guard, both of your opponent's legs are between your legs).

To perform this technique, put your feet together at your opponent's hip, and force him to the mat, face first. Tighten your legs and press his leg down across your body with his heel trapped in your elbow. from this position, arch your back and pull that elbow very tightly against his heel (Figs. 30–32).

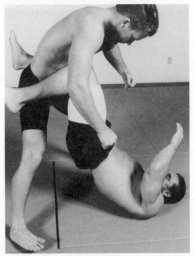

Figure 30

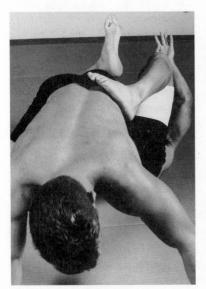

Figure 31

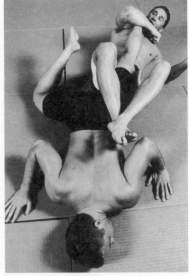

Figure 32

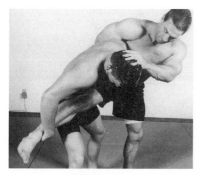

Figure 33

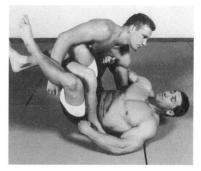

Figure 34

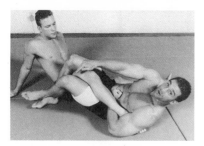

Figure 35

Achilles Lock

With this technique, pressure is applied on the Achilles tendon, which runs from the calf to the ankle. As illustrated, the lock is performed after a takedown (Figs. 33, 34), with your opponent's foot tucked under your armpit. It is important to

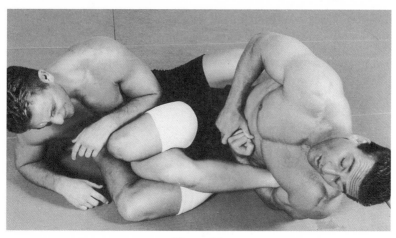

Figure 36

keep your opponent's leg tightly clamped between your thighs, and to press your wrist against the Achilles and lock your hands. The same principle we discussed with the rear choke also applies here. You are using the sharpest part of your forearm to apply pressure to the Achilles tendon. As you secure the hold, roll and arch your hips (Figs. 35, 36).

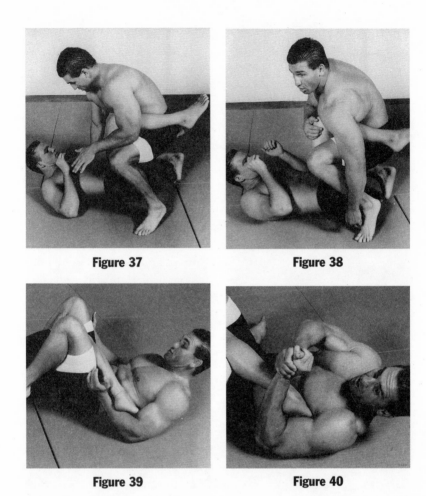

Figure 37   Figure 38

Figure 39   Figure 40

The Heel Hook

In my very first UFC fight, I faced Pat Smith. Smith, who is a tough fighter, swore before the event that he had a very high pain threshold and would to not tap out. Much to his surprise, however, I made him tap out with a simple heel hook. The heel hook is a good technique to perform when you are in your opponent's guard. To perform this technique, you split the guard (Figs. 37, 38) (more on splitting the guard in the next chapter), slide back and hook his heel between your wrist and armpit (Fig. 39). Next, lock your hands and turn your opponent's ankle across your chest (Fig. 40), keeping your thighs tight. As you might imagine, this causes great pain—enough to force even a tough man like Pat Smith to slap the canvas.

The Toe Submission

The toe submission is a variation of a simple and classic wrestling move. When a guy curls up real tight and you can't get to his neck or arm, fold one of your legs across the back of one of his knees (Fig. 41). Lock your foot under, behind your own knee, as you grab your opponent's foot with both hands. Grip the foot and rock back (Figs. 42, 43). This places excruciating pain on your opponent's knee.

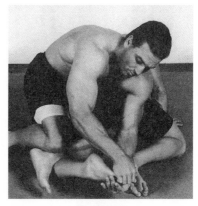

Figure 41

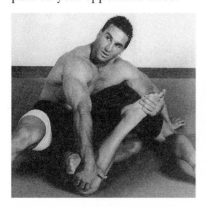

Figure 42

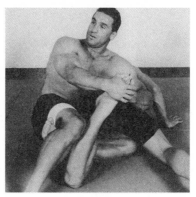

Figure 43

The Toe Hold

The toe hold, another simple but effective technique, can also be used when you split your opponent's guard and slip back. To apply a toe hold, simply lock your legs, grab the front of your opponents foot, and push. Be sure to push hard, arching your back, and using your abs, your

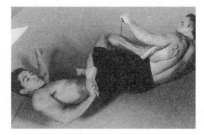

Figure 44

shoulders, and your arm. The pain this exerts on the knee is enough to bring a quick tap out from your opponent (Fig. 44).

Chapter 23

The Guard, the Mount, the Myth

Punishing, Escaping, and Winning

"Ken is a great fighter because of great preparation."

—Oleg Taktarov, Russian Sambo champion
and UFC 6 title-holder

It is a fact that most fights go to the ground. Fighting on the ground will undoubtedly involve time spent in either the guard or mount positions. In other words, in most fights you will have a chance to win or lose in either the guard or mount position.

As stated earlier, while in the guard position one fighter is on top and one below, face to face. The key factor in the guard is that the guy on the bottom has his legs wrapped around the guy on top. This gives the guy on the bottom a position of excellent control. The guy on top is said to be in his opponent's guard. In the mount, the guy on top has moved over his opponent's legs and is sitting happily on his opponent's chest, ready to bang away or attempt a submission hold. In general, it is better to be on the top in the guard and in the mount.

Some basic points I want to stress here are these: Some fighters in the UFC and elsewhere have tapped out once an opponent mounts them. They say the fight is over, that they don't want to get hit, and that there is no way to escape from the mount. That is a myth, pure garbage. You can escape from the mount as well as the guard. It's my personal belief that you should be willing to get hit once or twice when trying to escape from the mount. I have escaped from the mount several times myself, and I have had fighters escape from my mount. It does happen, and with greater frequency than many fighters assume. Let's now take a closer look at the guard and mount positions.

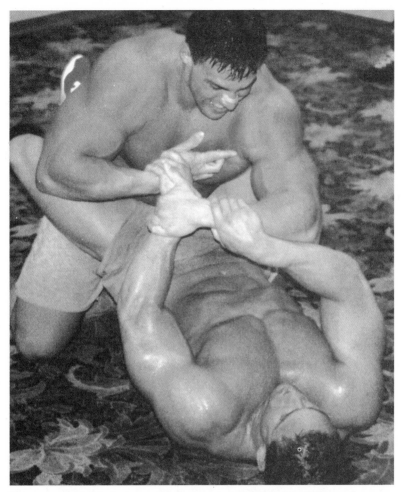

If your opponent is in your guard, you can usually control him and move to a choke or armbar. Here I am training with Dan Freeman (in my guard) a nationally recognized bodybuilder and a black belt in karate.

The Guard

When you are on the bottom, you can work for a leg choke or an armbar, as we've discussed. You are actually in control and in a good, solid position. If you want to leave the bottom position, maybe to scramble for a choke or to get back to your feet, here is a simple tip: grab your opponent's hands and pull them toward you (Fig. 1). His automatic reaction will be to pull back and away to resist your pull. When he does this, quickly release your hold and roll back away from your opponent (Fig. 2). You are now no longer on the bottom.

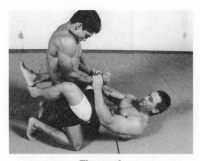

Figure 1

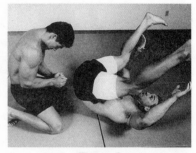

Figure 2

When you are on top, you can chip away with shots to the head and ribs and grind down your opponent, as I did in my second Superfight with Royce Gracie. When you punch to the ribs, aim for

the smallest rib, the one most vulnerable. Do not forget to dig your knuckles into the rib as your punch (Fig. 3). When your opponent moves his hand down to protect his rib, it's time to switch. Go for the ears and face. When he covers his ears and face, go back to the ribs. You will not knock anybody out this way or even

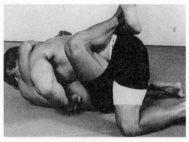

Figure 3

force a tap out, but over time this approach can steadily punish and weaken your opponent.

With most opponents, if you are on top in the guard position, you want to do one of two things. You want to move from the guard to the mount, by working your legs over the legs of your opponent. Or you want to split the guard, that is, separate his legs behind you, so you can slip into position for a submission hold. For example, I had to split the guard in my first UFC fight with Patrick Smith. Once I had

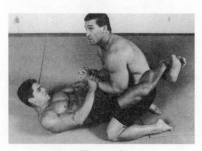

Figure 4

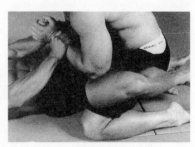

Figure 5

split the guard, I was able to rock back and apply a heel hook.

The best way to split the guard is to roll back and dig the tips of your elbows into your opponent's thighs (Figs. 4, 5). This causes extreme pain and will force him to move, usually separating his legs. (Most guys on the bottom will try to grab your hands so you can't strike them.)

Another way to split the guard is to plant a hard knee thrust at the base of your opponent's spine. To do this, separate his arms and pin them down at the elbow so he won't strike you. Rise to your knees, and slam a knee into his tailbone (Fig. 6). This produces pain and a loosening of the legs. Once the guard is split, you can quickly rock back, grab a leg, and your opponent is on his way

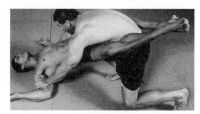

Figure 6

to tapping out. As you split the guard and move to a submission hold, be careful to maintain your balance. In that second or two between splitting and moving backward, your opponent can swing at you and attempt to apply a choke or submission hold of his own. Even though I stayed in Royce Gracie's guard for more than a half hour, in most fights I work the guard aggressively, either splitting the guard to go for a submission or maneuvering into the mounted position.

The Mount

If you are on top, congratula-tions. This is a good place to be. You have achieved a position of strength and dominance. Because your opponent's legs are behind you, he can't control you with them. With your superior position and angle, you have control.

Most guys when on the bot-tom will try to push your legs back so they can recapture you in their guard. When their hands go down to push, that gives you a clear opening to punch (Fig. 7).

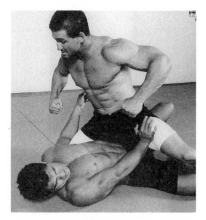

Figure 7

Remember the strike zone. Two or three quick punches connecting in the strike zone and you are on your way to victory, and your opponent

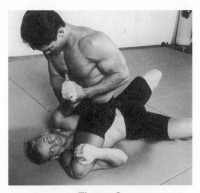

Figure 8

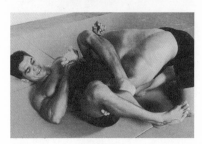

Figure 9

is on his way out. If for some reason the strikes are not landing, you can move forward, wrap a leg under his neck, and go for an armbar or leg lock (Figs. 8, 9).

Let's say, for example, that you are on the bottom and not the top. Don't give up. I repeat: don't give up! Yes, you want to move fast. Yes, you might get hit. So what are you waiting for, get going! You want to get out of this position as quickly as possible.

Here are some tactics for escape. You can bench press your opponent, pushing up on his chest, and getting a knee wedged up and between you. From this position, push or kick your opponent away (Fig. 10).

You can also blast a guy off of you by swinging your legs up and planting your heels into his chest. Just power him back off of you, and you will find yourself in a good position for a leg submission hold (Figs. 11–14). This move is most effective when your opponent has worked his way up toward your neck; it gives you more space in which to swing your legs up and more of an angle when you push him back.

You can also slip out the back door. This also works best when your opponent has positioned himself high onto your chest. To do this, grab his hands

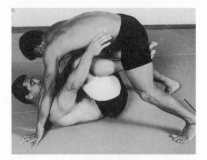

Figure 10

and swing your legs up (as you did in the previous movement), but instead of pushing your opponent back, curl low under your opponent and slip out the back door (Figs. 15, 16).

As a last resort, you can do a tuck and roll. The tuck and roll will expose you to the possibility of being locked by a rear choke, because your back will be turned to your opponent. However, if you move

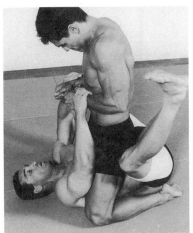

Figure 11

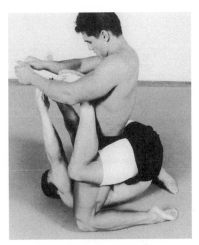

Figure 12

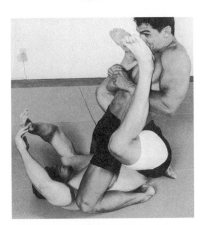

Figure 13

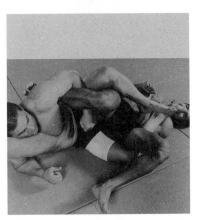

Figure 14

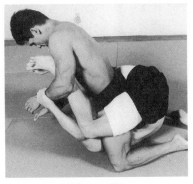

Figure 15

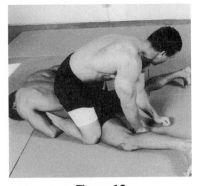

Figure 16

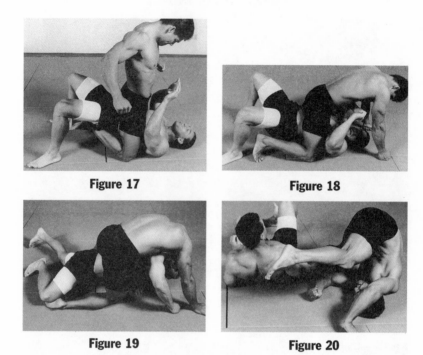

Figure 17   Figure 18

Figure 19   Figure 20

quickly and forcefully enough, there is a good chance you will get away. To begin the tuck and roll, bridge your back so that your opponent's weight moves forward, forcing him to post (or plant) his hands (Figs. 17, 18). Next, do a hip heist by flipping your hips and legs over so you are now in a crouched position (Fig. 19), then tuck your head and roll fast (Fig. 20). Do this as quickly as you can, or you will be snagged from behind.

Personally, I'd rather get caught in a submission hold trying to escape than to tap out because of the mere possibility that I might get punched a few times. If you enter a fight, enter it to win.

Chapter 24

Fight

Going into Battle

"Ken has so many qualities as a fighter. His strongest is his absolute belief that he will win, a belief that he instills in his fighters. So when you fight for Lion's Den, it is not a matter of whether you will win—it is just a matter of how you are going to do it."

—Guy Mezger, Lion's Den fighter.

Y ou've done your squats and crunches and push-ups. You've practiced your drills hundreds of times. You've sparred for long, tough hours, practicing your kicks, strikes, shoots, chokes, and submissions. You've eaten a sensible diet with lots of protein. You've hardened your body, calloused your mind. You are

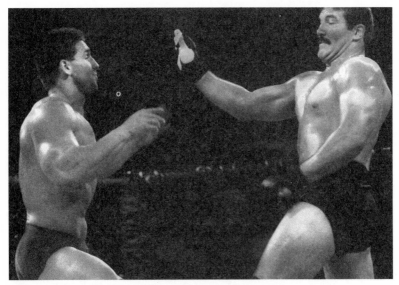

In my second Superfight with Dan Severn in Detroit, I looked for openings to throw a palm strike. *(Calixtro Romias photo)*

now ready to fight. Today is the big day. You will put it all together. You are going to war.

But if you haven't been in many fights, the idea of stepping onto a mat or into a dojo, let alone a UFC octagon, and engaging in real competition or combat can get you flustered. Don't let it. If you have worked hard, if you are prepared, you will do well. Be confident. Again: the fight is in the preparation. Part of that preparation is knowing your opponent. In a street fight, that's not easy. But even in a street fight or in a barroom brawl, you can get an advantage by comparing your opponent's size and strength to your own. Below are some things to look for.

If a guy is big and muscular, he is dangerous early but probably won't last long. He will usually be drained of energy pretty quickly, lose the power in his punch, allowing you to take him down and out. If you can stay with him for the first few minutes (assuming you are in shape), you will probably prevail. Big guys, as a rule, don't pace themselves—they usually go for a quick knock-out.

I was proud of how one of our Lion's Den fighters, Jerry Bohlander, did in his first UFC. He fought a huge guy, and a tough one, Scott Ferrozzo. Scott weighs more than 320 pounds, and Jerry weighs about 200 pounds. Jerry hung in there, fought with control, and let Scott wear himself down. Then, very quickly, Jerry found an opening and choked Scott, forcing him to tap out.

If you are fighting a guy with a tall, lean build, watch out for strikes. Those long arms and legs can reach out over a long distance and hurt you. Most top boxers and kickboxers are built this way. Their longer limbs allow them to punish you while trying to keep you from punishing them. With long limbs, they can also generate great velocity in their strikes and kicks. Patrick Smith has this kind of build. I knew he could throw some ferocious strikes and kicks, so I didn't let him. I took him to the ground. Don't try to battle "stand-up" with a Pat Smith. Instead, try to get in close, shoot in on him, take him to the ground, and neutralize his advantage. Obviously, if you have a Pat Smith build, tall or angular, use it to your advantage by throwing strikes to keep your opponent away from you.

If you are going against a wiry, compact opponent, don't count on wearing him down. You will need to use your power to your advantage and try to end the fight sooner rather than later. Pace yourself, do not exhaust yourself. When going after the smaller man, be aggressive, use your superior size. Be sure not to burn all the gas in your tank in the first thirty seconds of the fight.

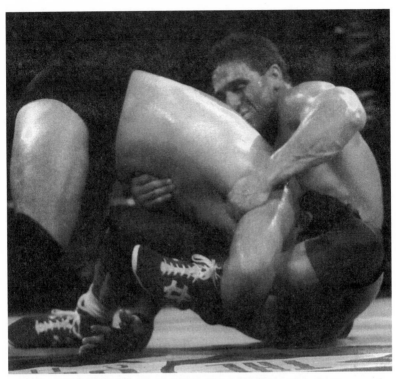

During most fights, there are changes in momentum. Hang in there and remain calm and tough. A few seconds after Severn had shot in on me in this photo, I had mounted him. *(Calixtro Romias photo)*

If you are fighting in a tournament and have some idea of who your opponent will be, get a sparring partner to imitate him. At Lion's Den, we have a variety of guest martial artists who spend time with us as we prepare for our fights. For instance, Maurice Smith has helped us with kicking and striking skills. In turn we've helped Maurice with grappling and submissions skills. If you can, your sparring should include a partner with similar size and technique as the guy you will be fighting. Before I fought Dan Severn, a really big guy with excellent wrestling experience, I worked out with Mike Radnov, a 260 pound personal trainer from Dallas and former top NCAA wrestler. Before I fought Kimo Leopaldo, another big guy with some martial arts background, I trained with Dan Freeman, a powerful, 270 pound black belt in karate who is a national-caliber bodybuilder.

On the day of a fight, make sure you eat enough and drink enough. Give yourself plenty of carbohydrates, but always allow two to three hours to digest that last meal or snack. Make sure you sip your water bottle and remain hydrated. Assuming your fight is in the late afternoon or at night, plan some activities, even if it's watching a movie. On the day of a fight, I usually get up pretty late, around 10:00 a.m. or so, and eat a big breakfast. Then I might take a walk, then watch a movie. I've watched *Braveheart*, and *Rocky*, and *The Terminator* on fight days. Watch something that grabs your attention, that might get your juices flowing a little. Be certain to stay relaxed. Do not dwell too much on the upcoming fight—enjoy a movie, read the paper, take a walk, watch a football game on TV, take a nap. If you are away from home, call your wife or girlfriend or your kids and chat for a while. This will help keep you calm and focused. If you find yourself getting queasy or hyper, try controlling your breathing. Take controlled, steady, even breaths. Then get back into the movie or book or back to your nap.

When I get to the arena for the fight, I usually settle in and relax until maybe an hour before the fight. Then I start slowly stretching every fiber of every limb. This is the time to start thinking about the fight to come, about how you are going to carry yourself. Check your breathing. Those controlled, steady breaths will really help you relax. About thirty minutes before a fight, I usually get a massage to help me loosen up even more. After the massage I might have a sparring partner go through a couple of moves. I may strike the focus mitts a few minutes to check my timing. In the hour before a fight, the main thing is to get loose and stretched, break a light sweat, and start mentally focusing on the fight to come.

Some guys have rituals they go through before a fight. They may tie and untie their shoelaces. They may go to the rest room and relieve themselves. They may drink a bottle of a sports drink. I have nothing against rituals and I have one myself: before all of my major fights, I have a moment of prayer with my dad, Bob. It helps me feel ready and confident. A ritual can help you feel comfortable in unfamiliar surroundings.

It has been said that you can go through a locker room before the fight and see who is going to win and who is going to lose. That's not entirely true, since I know some fighters who are pretty unglued in the locker room who still go out and fight like machines. However, this observation is valid to some extent. The guys who go through a pre-fight routine looking poised and cool tend to do well. Those who are pacing around, using the toilet every three minutes, looking jittery, tend not to do well. I think part of it is just feeling comfortable with yourself, and projecting that to everybody else. Even in the locker

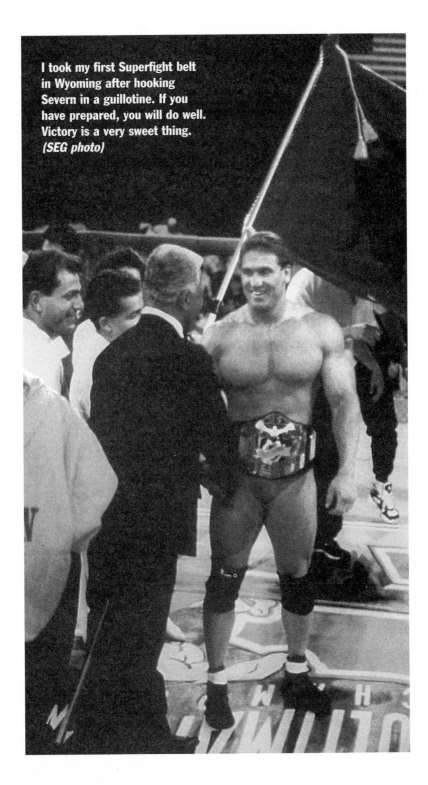

I took my first Superfight belt in Wyoming after hooking Severn in a guillotine. If you have prepared, you will do well. Victory is a very sweet thing. *(SEG photo)*

room, you are being checked out by a lot of people, including your opponent. Make sure you look like you have it all together, even if inside those butterflies are banging around in your stomach.

You should have a general game plan for the fight. Now, in the minutes before battle, is a good time to review it. In my second fight with Royce Gracie, I knew I wanted to take him to the ground and punish him without making any mistakes. With Kimo I knew I wanted to grapple with him and look for a leg submission. In my first fight with Dan Severn, I was looking for a chance to snag him in a guillotine choke because I knew he dropped his head as he went down to shoot. In the minutes before a fight, go through a list of opportunities you think may come up: the chance to strike, to grapple, or to choke. However, don't get too caught up in detail. A fight is a fluid thing, constantly changing and evolving. You have to be ready to adapt, to improvise, to overcome.

When you step into the octagon or onto the competition mat, decide whether or not you want to make eye contact with your opponent. I make eye contact if I can, because I like to look for fear, for excess energy, for the jitters. If you see any of these things, you have a hint of how your opponent is going to fight. If you do make contact, try to hold it. Let your opponent break it off. This gives you a minor psychological edge, but an edge nonetheless. Stay with an even, steady gaze. Give away nothing. Don't try to look like a maniac and don't try to look like a meditating monk. Just look firm and steady and determined. Let your eyes tell your opponent: "I am relaxed and prepared. I am ready for you." If you don't want to make eye contact, then don't make it. But I suggest you either make eye contact and hold it, or don't make it at all. Don't glance at a guy, catch his eye, then turn away. This is a sign of weakness.

Be aware of your body language. Keep your chin up and your chest out. Don't glance around and check out the cameras or the judges or the spectators. Look strong and steady.

When the fight starts, let your adrenaline and instincts propel you, push you off. Try not to let them overwhelm you. You might be fighting for a long time, so don't get burned out in an adrenaline rush. As a fight continues, watch your breathing. If you start breathing too fast, you will use up too much energy. Try to remain charged but under control. You must be able to think quickly and clearly. If the fight goes well in the early stages, fine. If it doesn't, don't panic. I'll say it again: Do Not Panic!

In most fights, and in most athletic competitions in general, there are changes in momentum. It is rare for one person or team to dominate from start to finish. There are usually ebbs and flows, highs and lows. In a fight, you must hang tough even if things shift. In that UFC fight in San Juan, Jerry Bohlander wanted to take Scott Ferrozzo to the ground in the middle of the octagon. Instead, Ferrozzo charged him and pinned him against the fence like a bug on a windshield. But Jerry did not panic. He was patient, and he won the fight.

In your fight, be aggressive, but be patient and be confident. Look for the opportunities. This is where the running, crunches, and squats you've done in the previous weeks pay off. If a match drags on, and you've done your conditioning, your preparation, you can take a lot of encouragement from the fact that you can outlast your opponent. If you end up in a siege, with a guy hanging onto you for dear life, sometimes outlasting him is all you can do. Make sure when you step into competition that you have the conditioning that will let you prevail in a long fight.

In most fights, there comes a moment of opportunity. This is especially true with my system, where the whole objective is to find a chance to apply a choke hold or clamp a lock on an opponent's arm or leg. When that opportunity comes don't hesitate, seize it. Pursue it with everything you have. Whether it's a choke or lock or a chance to strike with finishing power, do it. It is a living example of the old phrase about smelling blood. When you get a whiff that you can finish the fight, it's got to be all out. You must go for it despite getting hit or kicked. In my UFC fight against Patrick Smith, he landed some elbows and kicks on me as I planted in my heel hook. The strikes took a toll. They hurt, but I did not release my hold. I weathered the storm and Smith tapped out.

The ability to finish a tough no-holds-barred fight separates the great fighters from good ones, the boys from the men. The great fighters can do more than hang with guys indefinitely. They know how to finish. Again, you find this in a lot of sports. It's the football team that recovers a fumble on the 20 and pushes in for a touchdown. It's the tennis player who gets into a tie breaker and revs into a higher gear. It's the runner who sees the finish line and pushes himself to lunge ahead of the field. Some might call it the killer instinct. I just think it's part of being a competitor.

Anybody who fights at a high level, and fights frequently, is going to get beat. In the octagon, you can either tap out or John McCarthy, the referee, can stop the fight. How do you know when to tap out, to surrender with dignity? Oleg Taktarov has told me he would never tap

out; he says it is just part of his Russian fighting heritage. I see it differently, however. If you are not able to defend yourself and you are
in immediate danger of suffering a major injury, such as torn ligaments, tap out and preserve your body. You can come back to fight
another day. On the other hand, if your opponent has achieved a superior position, and you can still defend yourself, by all means do so. In
one of the UFC events, a fighter tapped out simply because his opponent achieved a mount position on him. That's not my style. First of
all, as we have discussed earlier, the mount isn't a hopeless position.
Yes, you may get hit. But, if you go into the UFC thinking you won't
be hit a few times, you are in denial. You will get hit and if you can't
accept it, don't sign up. Even in the mount position there are ways to
defend yourself, ways to escape. It has been done. Hang tough and
show some heart.

If you are getting choked, there comes a point where the choke is
sunk in and you can't get out of it. You know this when you begin to
lose consciousness. The important thing to remember when in a
choke is this: stay calm, resist, defend, and try to escape. This is not
easy, and it takes experience before you can know the point at which
you can still launch an escape and the point where you should tap out.
And it's a funny thing with chokes. When one is set or being set, most
guys get a powerful, basic urge to give up. The only time I have
tapped out in the UFC was when Royce Gracie wrapped a choke on
me. Looking back, I should have resisted with more ferocity. Instead,
I pounded the canvas. We all live and learn.

After a fight, win or lose, Lion's Den fighters show respect to their
opponents. I usually shake hands or give my opponent a bear hug.
Don't make any excuses for a loss. Give the credit where it belongs,
to the guy who beat you. Inwardly, you may know you didn't fight well
or made mistakes. You may have gone through a monster preliminary
fight that left you bruised and battered, while your opponent's preliminary fight may have been a joke. Like life itself, competitive fighting is not always fair. That's simply the way it is. You may chew it all
over later with your manager, coach, wife, or good friends. But excuses are not something you need to share in the moments after a fight.
The period immediately after a fight says a lot about a fighter. Win or
lose, do it with dignity.

Later, take some time to go through the fight and explore what you
did well, and what you could have done better. Make a mental note of
your opponent's strengths and weaknesses. There is a chance you will
face him again someday. Talk about the fight with your coach, man-

ager, or other fighters. Maybe they noticed something you didn't. Don't be arrogant or defensive about this. It is always important that you be open to feedback. That is how you are going to progress.

At some point, though, whether you have won or lost, you need to put the fight behind you. Rededicate yourself to your training, to preparations for your next fight. Look ahead. If you lost your last fight, work for redemption, as I did against Royce Gracie. If you won, work to build your skills and reputation even further.

Becoming an outstanding fighter in any martial art is not a quick and easy process. You will suffer. You will lose. You will hurt. But if you continue, and you learn, and you have heart, you will eventually triumph. You will become a champion.

I'm glad you joined us here at the Lion's Den. I hope these lessons help you the next time you face an aggressive drunk or step into realistic martial arts competition. Good luck, and stay hungry. Take pride in what you do, in who you are, and never, never stop learning.

Afterword

There have been many changes in the life of Ken Shamrock since his Superfight with Dan Severn in Detroit.

In June 1996, Bob Shamrock met in Los Angeles with Rorion Gracie. The two discussed staging a rematch between Ken Shamrock and Royce Gracie. Shamrock, with friend Jay Wilton, proposed the Shamrocks and Gracies each side put up $2 million, with $1 million toward production costs and $1 million toward the purse. The Gracies declined, saying they did not have sufficient financing.

Shamrock fought in the UFC's Ultimate Ultimate tournament in late 1996 and beat kickboxer Brian Johnston. It would be his final fight in the UFC.

In February 1997, Shamrock signed a contract with the World Wrestling Federation, a major pro-wrestling company. Shamrock anguished over the decision for days. He wanted to continue fighting in the UFC, building his legend as one of the best no-holds-barred warriors in modern times. But Shamrock also felt a need to provide for his family's future. The WWF contract, far richer than anything the UFC might provide, offered that opportunity. In the end, Shamrock decided to sign with the WWF.

He will continue to operate the Lion's Den, and the Lodi-based dojo will continue to develop fighters for reality fighting events all over the world. Bob Shamrock closed his group home for boys in late 1996 to devote more time to building and expanding the Lion's Den.

Shamrock's older brothers, Richie and Robbie Kilpatrick, continue to do well. Both live in the Napa area. Richie is attending college, working toward a degree in telecommunications and holding down a full-time job. Robbie works as a concrete finisher and is employed part-time at a fitness center. He works out regularly at the Lion's Den and hopes of becoming a no-holds-barred fighter.

On July 12, 1997, Tina and Ken Shamrock became the proud parents of a baby girl, Fallon Marie Shamrock. She is a healthy and beautiful child.

Just a few weeks before Fallon's birth, the Shamrocks moved to the ranch in the rolling hills east of Lodi, near the town of Clements. The spread includes more than twenty acres and a spacious yellow ranch house.

It is a quiet place, a place with a creek that meanders through grassy, golden fields dotted with towering oaks.

It will be a good place to raise a family.

Ken Shamrock
Career Highlights

December 7, 1996, Birmingham, AL: Shamrock, unleashing a ferocious flurry of strikes, forces kickboxing champion Brian Johnston to tap out after five minutes in the Ultimate Fighting Champion's Ultimate Ultimate tournament. Shamrock breaks his hand during the fight, however, and is unable to progress to the semi-finals of the competition.

May 17, 1996, Detroit, MI: In a controversial split decision, judges award Dan Severn, a Greco-Roman wrestling champion, the Superfight belt after Severn and Shamrock go the distance in a largely defensive contest.

February 16, 1996, Puerto Rico: Shamrock beats Kimo Leopoldo, a 270-pound taekwondo fighter, in UFC VIII and retains his Superfight belt.

September 8 1995, New York: Shamrock retains his UFC Superfight belt after dominating Russian Sambo champion Oleg Taktarov.

July 14, 1995, Wyoming: Shamrock claims the UFC Superfight crown with a quick victory over Severn. Shamrock uses a guillotine choke to force Severn's tap-out.

April 7, 1995, Charlotte, NC: In the longest UFC bout ever, Shamrock controls and bludgeons reigning champion Royce Gracie for 36 minutes and 6 seconds avenging an earlier loss to the ju-jitsu champion. Gracie drops out of UFC competition after the beating and Shamrock, by default, progresses to another Superfight battle.

December 16 & 17, 1994, Tokyo: Shamrock prevails over a group of the world's finest martial artists to become the first-ever King of Pancrase. Opponents in the Pancrase tournament include Alex Cook, Maurice Smith, Masa Funaka, and Manabu Yamada.

September 9, 1994, Charlotte, NC: Shamrock beats Christoph Leininger, a U.S. judo champion, and Felix Mitchell, a kickboxer, to win a place in the finals of UFC III. Shamrock withdraws after Gracie forfeits his semi-final match because of exhaustion.

July 24, 1994, Tokyo: In a Pancrase match, Shamrock uses a submission hold to beat Dutch fighting champion Bas Ruten in sixteen minutes, forty-two seconds.

November 12, 1993, Denver, CO: In the first ever Ultimate Fighting Championships, Shamrock defeats taekwondo champion Patrick Smith with a heel hook and loses to Royce Gracie in the semi-final match.

November 8, 1993, Tokyo: Shamrock chokes out Pancrase fighter Yusuke Fuke in forty-four seconds.

September 21, 1993, Tokyo: In his first appearance for the Pancrase hybrid Wrestling organization, Shamrock defeats Masa Funaki in six minutes, fifteen seconds using a choke hold.

1992, Tokyo: Shamrock becomes one of the first *gaijin*, or foreigner, to become a champion in Japanese submission fighting.

January 1990, North Carolina: Shamrock wins his third Toughman competition in Hickory, North Carolina, by knock-out. He had earlier won Toughman contests in Mooresville, North Carolina and Redding, California.

Glossary

Battlecade, Inc.: The company which created and produces Extreme Fighting, a pay-per-view event. Battlecade is backed by General Media International, which publishes *Penthouse* magazine.

Blown up: Exhausted, spent.

Bridge: To arch the back and neck from a prone position, often to roll an opponent.

Calloused: When a part of the body has been roughened to absorb punishment with little pain or damage. Also refers to mental toughness achieved to absorb pain and continue fighting.

Dojo: The building where training and sparring take place. A dojo can be as elaborate as a temple or a simple as a bare room. Ken Shamrock's dojo, Lion's Den, is a converted concrete warehouse with few amenities.

Duck walk: A conditioning exercise in which fighters bend their knees and stride forward, their buttocks only inches from the floor. The duck walk builds leg strength and balance; Lion's Den fighters use it to prepare for shooting in on opponents.

Extreme Fighting: A reality fighting event shown on pay-per-view television.Unlike the Ultimate Fighting Championship, Extreme Fighting includes rounds, called "phases," as well as weight divisions. The first event was held on November 18 1995 at a movie studio in Wilmington, North Carolina. The second event was staged on a Mohawk Indian reservation in Canada. After the event, five fighters and three officials were arrested and detained by Mohawk peace keepers on charges of engaging in an illegal prizefight, the U.S. equivalent of a misdemeanor.

Fishhook: To slip a thumb or finger into the opponent's mouth in order to tear at the soft tissue of the lips or cheeks; banned in the UFC and Pancrase.

Gassed: Roughly the same as blown up; exhausted and vulnerable.

Guard: A position in which one fighter in on his back and the other is lodged over him. In the guard position, the man on the bottom has his legs wrapped around the fighter in the superior position; this allows the man below to achieve a high level of defensive control.

Mount: A position similar to the guard, except that the man below does not have his legs wrapped around his opponent and therefore lacks the defensive control afforded by the guard. The mount is a favorable position for the man on top, who can rain blows down on his opponent. Though the mount is a difficult spot for the man below, it does not spell automatic defeat. Skilled fighters can often curl up in defensive posture to avoid punishment and eventually spin or slide out.

NHB, No Holds Barred: Fights with few if any rules.

Octagon: The eight-sided fighting arena used in the Ultimate Fighting Championship; conceived by John Milius, a creative consultant for the event and a prominent screenwriter.

Pancrase Hybrid Wrestling: A popular fighting organization in Japan that holds fights featuring open-hand strikes, kicks and submissions holds. Under Pancrase rules, there are no head butts or closed-fist strikes. A fighter in trouble can prompt a restart by grabbing the ropes. (Ken Shamrock won the first Pancrase championship tournament in 1995, claiming the title "King of Pancrase.")

Pancration: A hand-to-hand combat event developed by the ancient Greeks. Pancration included striking, kicking and grappling skills. It was the most popular offering of the early Olympics, drawing more spectators than either boxing or wrestling.

Palm strike: In Pancrase and some other fighting events, closed-fist strikes are prohibited. The preferred blow is the palm strike, delivered with either a forehand or backhand movement.

Post: Planting a leg or arm to gain stability. When fighters throw a punch, they typically post their lead leg.

Reality fighting: The Ultimate Fighting Championship and Extreme Fighting are both examples of reality fighting, full-contact martial arts competitions whose outcomes are not pre-determined. Scramble: In grappling, fighters scramble when neither has a dominant position and each fighter is working furiously to achieve an advantage.

SEG: Semaphore Entertainment Group, based in New York City, is the company that owns and produces the Ultimate Fighting Championship.

Shuck: To fend off or push away a strike or kick.

Schooled: Dominated, badly beaten. When a fighter is quickly and convincingly defeated, he has been schooled.

Shoot, shootfighting: A shoot is an explosive move toward an opponent, low and hard, with the goal of taking him to the mat. Shootfighting is a brand of martial art that emphasizes grappling and punching.

Squat: A basic and simple exercise to build strength in the legs. The fighter bends his knees and lowers his body, keeping his back straight, then rises. The squat is a basic exercise for submission fighting.

Submission Fighting: The style of fighting, popularized by Ken Shamrock, stressing chokes and joint locks. Known as submissions because the goal is to make the opponent submit, usually by tapping out. The lineage of heritage of submission fighting extends to the pancration events in Greece.

Sunk in: When a joint lock or choke is firmly in place.

Tap out: To submit or give up. Performed by tapping or slapping the mat with the hand.

Ultimate Fighting Championship: One of the most popular events on pay-per-view television, the Ultimate Fighting Championship has drawn unprecedented attention to the martial arts in the United States. The first UFC was staged in Denver in November 1993. Founders included Art Davie, a Los Angeles adman and former boxer, and Rorion Gracie, whose family practices Brazilian ju-jitsu. Gracie had also worked as a technical advisor for several movies, including "Lethal Weapon." Along with other investors, they formed W.O.W. promotions, for War of the Worlds. They staged the first UFC in a partnership with the Semaphore Entertainment Group, a New York-based firm specializing in cable television productions. Davie, Gracie and other initial investors eventually sold their interests to SEG, owned by Robert Meyrowitz.